Proceedings of the Fifth Annual Conference of the British Association for Biological Anthropology and Osteoarchaeology

Edited by

Sonia R. Zakrzewski
Margaret Clegg

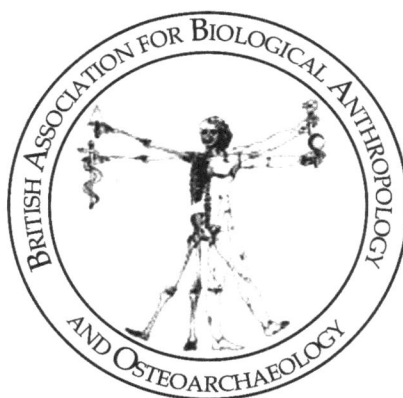

BAR International Series 1383
2005

Published in 2016 by
BAR Publishing, Oxford

BAR International Series 1383

*Proceedings of the Fifth Annual Conference of the British Association for Biological
Anthropology and Osteoarchaeology*

ISBN 978 1 84171 823 1

BAR Publishing is the trading name of British Archaeological Reports (Oxford) Ltd.
British Archaeological Reports was first incorporated in 1974 to publish the BAR
Series, International and British. In 1992 Hadrian Books Ltd became part of the BAR
group. This volume was originally published by Archaeopress in conjunction with
British Archaeological Reports (Oxford) Ltd / Hadrian Books Ltd, the Series principal
publisher, in 2005. This present volume is published by BAR Publishing, 2016.

Printed in England

BAR
PUBLISHING

BAR titles are available from:

BAR Publishing
122 Banbury Rd, Oxford, OX2 7BP, UK
EMAIL   info@barpublishing.com
PHONE   +44 (0)1865 310431
FAX   +44 (0)1865 316916
www.barpublishing.com

Contents

Introduction

Margaret Clegg & Sonia R. Zakrzewski

Centre for the Archaeology of Human Origins
Dept of Archaeology, University of Southampton,
Highfield, Southampton, SO17 1BF

This volume represents the first publication of the conference proceedings of the British Association for Biological Anthropology and Osteoarchaeology and consists of a sample of the papers and posters presented at the Association's Fifth annual conference Since its inception the Association has striven to include all aspects of research within Osteoarchaeology and the wider field of Biological Anthropology.. The first conference was held in Birmingham, in 1999, and included sessions entitled "Planning, Excavation, Processing and Curation of Human Skeletal Remains" and "Human Growth and Reproduction". More recently, the conferences have included sessions which concentrated upon aspects of palaeopathology and comparative primate morphology and behaviour. These conferences have been notable for demonstrating the breadth and diversity in research within the field of biological anthropology, both within the UK and from further afield. The conferences have been highly successful at developing osteoarchaeology within Britain, through sharing the research being undertaken with a wider audience, and from developing British standards for the recording of human skeletal remains (Brickley & McKinley 2004)

The fifth conference was held in Southampton in 2003 and was attended by over 120 people. The sessions included in the conference ranged from "Agency of Osteology in Social Archaeology", through chemistry in osteoarchaeology, primates and hominid evolution and mummies and their mummification to "Fragmentation of the Body: Comestibles, Compost or Customary Rite?". Most podium sessions included linked poster presentations. This publication therefore presents a representative sample of the material presented within the general themes of the conference sessions.

Although this publication forms the first volume of the conference proceedings to be published, it is intended that this will become the normal occurrence. As a result this volume tries to set the standards for publication of the association's conference proceedings by having all the papers submitted subjected to full peer-review. As editors, we have been strict in following the requirements and comments made by the reviewers, and hence we feel that the following papers are all of a high standard. It is noteworthy that the papers themselves are written by a wide variety of researchers, from postgraduate students to Professors, and also include some from researchers outside academia. The volume is organised into four loose themes.

The first theme, consisting of the first five papers, concerns the taphonomic aspects of the study of osteoarchaeology, and these papers provide some cautionary notes for researchers to remember. Bello points out the importance of considering all the factors that might influence the preservation of bones at a site and argues that one should not simply assume that a lack of smaller bones indicates such practices as secondary burial. She further reminds us that under-representation of particular age classes may not be due to differential burial, but rather due to taphonomic processes acting, for example, on immature bones She outlines the interactions between taphonomy, burial practices and anatomy upon skeletal preservation. Loe and Cox discuss the importance of surface features and modification of bone at or around the time of death. They describe a protocol for recording such features and suggest that any exploration of bone fracture and fragmentation should consider the relationships with such features. White takes us through the processes involved in soft tissue preservation and gives a clear and wide ranging insight into this topic. Beckett and Cherryson provide two closely linked papers that remind us that monumental tombs and graveyards are not static through time, but instead that they have been continually disturbed through such factors as re-use. Beckett discusses the processes involved in the reuse of this space in terms of the categorisation processes acting in the minds of past populations. Cherryson, by contrast, suggests that the level of disturbance may inform us regarding the process of urbanisation in society.

The next three papers fall into a general category of osteological report, and contain details of interesting sites and samples which merit further research. These range from the Neolithic site described by Leach through Norton Priory and the pathologies encountered in a medieval monastery found by Boylston and Ogden to the post medieval tallow Hill site described by Ogden and co-workers.

The next three papers provide case studies which link research concepts with the skeletal and mummy record to provide theoretically challenging discussion. Gill-Robinson surveys the current state of knowledge regarding bog bodies within

Europe. She shows that the number of bodies is less than that sometimes suggested in the literature and describes traditional and novel methods for obtaining further data from these bodies. Using an example from Florida (Wendover), Hamlin shows how preservation of both skeletal and material culture can inform our views of gender roles in the past. This rare site allows a glimpse of past practices that earlier researchers did not consider. The final paper in this section, by Barrientos and co-workers, looks at changing perspectives of the same material over time and how a different view point radically changes the opinions of the researchers. The case study presented here derives from South America and concerns evidence for the first population and colonisation processes.

The last theme contains the more technical osteological studies, wherein the skeletal material is challenged for its potential to reveal further information or ideas about past and current populations. Using a Neolithic sample from Orkney, Bernal and co-workers show that statistical analysis of morphological variation can allow us to determine whether the variation discovered in assemblages from the same geographic region is most likely to be the result of genetic drift or distinct biological differences between the samples. Storm and Knüsel discuss the usefulness of the assessment of fluctuating asymmetry within the skeletal record and demonstrate how metric analysis can pinpoint variation that might otherwise be overlooked. Gapert and Last explore the occiput's role in sex and ethnic determination. They determine the most reliable markers for such analyses. Finally, Gowland and Chamberlain incorporate Bayesian statistics into a traditional pubic symphyseal ageing method in order to obtain demographic profiles of past populations.

We hope that these papers will demonstrate the diversity and depth of research in biological anthropology presented at the conference. Many other papers and posters were presented, and so the papers included here should be viewed as simply a selection of those presented.

Literature Cited

Brickley, M & J McKinley (2004) Guidelines to the Standards for Recording Human Remains. IFA Paper Number 7. IFA/BABAO Publication.
http://www.soton.ac.uk/~babao/HumanremainsFINAL.pdf

The reciprocal effects of taphonomy, funerary practices and anatomical features on the state of preservation of human remains.

Taphonomy and state of preservation of human remains.

Silvia Bello

Palaeontology Department, The Natural History Museum
Cromwell Road
London
SW7 5BD
s.bello@nhm.ac.uk

Abstract

This paper aims to distinguish the preservation patterns relating to the anatomical characteristics of human bones and the secondary effects of taphonomical processes resulting from burial practices and/or cultural activities. Understanding the impact of environmental and/or cultural factors on the state of preservation of human skeletons is crucial for optimising the information to be gained from the skeletal remains of historic and prehistoric populations. Differences in the state of preservation and/or representation of bones, individuals or a specific class of individuals may be alternatively ascribed to taphonomic processes, cultural practices or anatomical features of the skeleton. The impact of these extrinsic and intrinsic factors on the preservation of human remains was determined by analysing four osteological human samples, and the effect of differential patterns of preservation on anthropological studies are discussed. Differing patterns of preservation have been seen to directly influence the type and quantity of information that may be derived from osteoarchaeological samples.

Key words: Taphonomy, burial practices, preservation pattern, human bones.

Introduction

The factors determining the state of preservation of human remains may be intrinsic and extrinsic to the bones. Intrinsic factors are defined by anatomical features such as size, shape, density, mineral and water content, as well as the state of health, sex and biological age of the individual. Henderson (1987) recognised three main categories of extrinsic factor: the environment of the site (climate, topography and geology), the nature of the local flora and fauna, and human activity. Determining the nature of the extrinsic factors in case of burials can be difficult, as natural taphonomic processes may be strictly connected to funerary practices and burial structures. Humans are the only species that pays attention to their dead, acting in accordance with the criteria and cultural expression of the period, which goes beyond the mere necessity of simply disposing of the bodies. Remains may be found in single, collective or multiple burials, in funerary structures, under floors of houses or as scavenged discards. They may be complete skeletons, broken remains, or cremation residues. Much of this variability comes as a result of human activity, but some also results from natural post-mortem changes, normally referred to as taphonomic processes.

It is important to understand the part played by taphonomy, burial practice and intrinsic anatomical features in determining the state of preservation of human remains in order to recognise the processes responsible for the formation of an assemblage, and to identify specific patterns of bone modification revealing intentional human activities. For example, the relative abundance of specific bones, such as the skull, and the under-representation of others, such as the bones of the hands and feet, has often been associated with secondary burial. This conclusion should, however, be mediated by the intrinsic characteristics of smaller and less mineralised bones, which often determine their under-representation irrespective of the characteristics of the site. Indeed the under- and over-representation of specific bones in an assemblage could be the result of the normal reaction of these bones to the environment of the site and its natural and/or artificial characteristics (Bello & Andrews accepted paper a). Funeral and burial practices can also select a portion of the population according to biological (sex, age, family relationship) and/or social criteria. Selective burial or non-burial of all or parts of individuals belonging to a particular subgroup of the population, as well as the use of differing burial structures for different subgroups, will result in a bias in the palaeodemographical reconstruction of the original population (Bello et al. 2002; Margerison & Knüsel 2002). The exclusion of the new-born and the old, who may not be recognised as active members of the community, is well-known from historical periods (Dedet et al. 1991; Perrin 2000; Tranoy 2000). However, this under-representation of subadults, and especially the very young children, could be related to intrinsic factors leading to non-preservation of less-mineralised and smaller immature bones.

Table 1: List of the osteoarchaeological collections studied.

Site	Location	Type	Period	NMI	Demography
St Maximin	France	Modern cemetery	14th-18th century	3	2 adult females 1 adult male
		Late Medieval cemetery	12th-13th century	79	34 subadults 14 adult females 12 adult females 9 adults
		Early Medieval cemetery	6th-7th century	7	1 subadult 2 adult females 3 adult males 1 adult
St Estève le Pont	France	Cemetery	8th Century	84	32 subadults 29 adult females 20 adult males 3 adults
Observance	France	Plague Pit	1722	179	51 subadults 58 adult females 59 adult males 11 adults
Spitalfields	UK	Crypt	1729-1857	357	37 subadult females 42 subadult males 139 adult females 139 adult males

What effect does differential states of preservation of osseous material have on anthropological studies? Differing patterns of preservation directly influence the type and quantity of information that may be derived from osteoarchaeological samples. Non-fragmentary and well preserved bones allow fine osteometrical and palaeopathological analyses while the complete representation of all individual classes guarantees correct palaeodemographical reconstruction.

This paper outlines the way in which taphonomy, burial practices and anatomical features are inter-related in determining the state of preservation of human osteoarchaeological collections, and shows how different patterns of preservation of osseous remains can influence the anthropological interpretations of historic and prehistoric populations.

Material and Method

The analysis has been focused on four human osteological samples from different funerary contexts (table 1).

Age at death for the skeletons found at St Maximin, St. Estève le Pont and Observance was estimated using macroscopic analysis of dental markers (Miles 1963; Lamandin 1978; Ubelaker 1989), long bone markers (Fazekas & Kosa 1978; Birkner 1980; White & Folkens 1991; Buikstra & Ubelaker 1994; Scheuer & Black 2000) and signs of degenerative reactions in the bones (Stewart 1957). Sex determination was based on observation of the pelvis using the methods proposed by Genovés (1959),

Stewart (1979), Hoyme (1984) and Iscan (1989). Individuals' sex and age at Spitalfields sample were derived directly from coffin plates and confirmed by historical sources where possible (according to Molleson and Cox 1993).

The state of preservation of the human bones was evaluated using three preservation indices: the Anatomical Preservation Index (API; Bello 2001), the Bone Representation Index (BRI, Dodson and Wexlar 1979) and the Qualitative Bone Index (QBI; Bello 2001).

The Anatomical Preservation Index (API; Bello 2001) expresses the ratio between the score of preservation (i.e. the percentage of bone preserved) for each single bone and the skeleton's total anatomical number of bones. The preservation scores were arranged in six classes (table 2). Well preserved bones (WPB) were defined as those having a preservation score of more than 50% (classes 4, 5 and 6), and well preserved skeletons (WPS) as those having more than 50% of their bones well preserved.

Intra-observer and inter-observer errors were tested using a t-test for paired observations. The preservation scores were estimated by the author and a second researcher on 34 osseous remains all coming from a single skeleton. Both the intra- and the inter-observer errors produced a t-score very close to 1, showing that there was neither a significant difference between the two scores given at two different times by the same observer nor between the scores awarded to the same specimen by two different observers.

Table 2: Preservation scores used to evaluate the anatomical Preservation Index (API)

Class of preservation	% of bone preserved
Class 1	0%
Class 2	1-24 %
Class 3	25-49%
Class 4	50-74%
Class 5	75-99%
Class 6	100%

The Bone Representation Index (BRI; Dodson & Wexlar 1979) measures the frequency of each bone in the sample. It is the ratio between the actual number of bones removed during excavation and the theoretical number of bones that should have been present according to the Minimum Number of Individuals (MNI) in the sample:

$$BRI = 100 \times \Sigma \text{ No. obs. / No. theor.}$$

Well-represented bones (WRB) were defined as those having a representation in the sample of more than 50% and well represented skeletons (WRS) as those having more than 50% of their bones represented.

The state of preservation of cortical surfaces was evaluated using the Qualitative Bone Index (QBI; Bello 2001), being the ratio between the sound cortical surface and the damaged surface of each single bone. The state of preservation of cortical surfaces was grouped into six qualitative classes (table 3). Well preserved cortical surfaces (BWPCS) were defined as those having a cortical surface preservation score of more than 50% (classes 4, 5 and 6) and skeletons with well preserved cortical surfaces (SWPCS) as those having more than 50% of their bones with well preserved cortical surfaces.

Table 3: Preservation scores used to evaluate the Qualitative Bone Index (QBI).

Class of preservation	% of sound cortical surface
Class 1	0%
Class 2	1-24 %
Class 3	25-49%
Class 4	50-74%
Class 5	75-99%
Class 6	100%

The intra-observer error produced a t-score very close to 1, indicating that there was no significant difference between two assessments taken at two times by the same observer. The inter-observer error produced a t-score of 0.832 with an associated p-value of 0.794, showing that there was no significant difference between the scores awarded to the same specimen by two different observers.

Results

1. Extrinsic factors
1.1 Site characteristics

The frequency of well preserved bones, qualitatively well preserved bones and the BRI values were calculated for subadult and adult individuals in the four studied samples (Table 4).

Table 4: Frequencies of Well-preserved bones, BRI and Bones with Well Preserved Cortical Surfaces in the samples observed.

	Subadult	Adult	Whole
% Well Preserved Bones			
St. Maximin			41.4
6th-7th Cemetery			35.3
12th-13th Cemetery	40.5	42.3	41.4
14th-18th Cemetery			79.4
St. Estève	26.3	59.6	46.9
Observance	48.7	67.3	62.0
Spitalfields	43.5	61.2	57.1
BRI			
St. Maximin			55.8
6th-7th Cemetery			55.9
12th-13th Cemetery	56.2	55.5	55.8
14th-18th Cemetery			92.2
St. Estève	50.2	83.0	70.5
Observance	65.7	80.3	76.2
Spitalfields	58.0	76.7	72.4
% Bones with Well Preserved Cortical Surfaces			
St. Maximin			90.4
6th-7th Cemetery			96.9
12th-13th Cemetery	92.8	88.3	90.5
14th-18th Cemetery			95.7
St. Estève	48.0	69.1	62.8
Observance	69.2	88.2	81.9
Spitalfields	91.1	96.6	95.6

The remains from St. Maximin and St. Estève le Pont cemeteries were generally more poorly preserved than those from Observance and Spitalfields (Table 5). The better state of preservation observed at Observance and Spitalfields is probably related to the environmental characteristics of these sites which guaranteed good protection for the bones: a dip pit in the case of Observance site and a Crypt in the case of Spitalfields site.

Table 5: Statistically significant differences in frequency of well preserved bones and BRI values evaluated for the 4 studied collections.

Differences in the frequencies of well preserved bones (API)

St. Maximin / Observance	$\chi^2 = 88.229$	p < 0.0001
St. Maximin / Spitalfields	$\chi^2 = 62.212$	p < 0.0001
St. Maximin / St. Estève I	$\chi^2 = 4.556$	p = 0.0327
St. Estève / Observance	$\chi^2 = 52.993$	p< 0.0001
St. Estève / Spitalfields	$\chi^2 = 30.774$	p< 0.0001

Differences in BRI values

St. Maximin / St. Estève	$\chi^2 = 23.764$	p < 0.0001
St. Maximin / Observance	$\chi^2 = 58.934$	p < 0.0001
St. Maximin / Spitalfields	$\chi^2 = 46.407$	p < 0.0001
St. Estève / Observance	$\chi^2 = 4.941$	p < 0.0262

The three areas at St. Maximin site present differing patterns of preservation, with the Modern cemetery having the highest frequencies of well preserved bones and the highest BRI values (these figures might have been biased by the scarcity of human remains in the Modern and Early Medieval cemeteries). While the state of preservation of cortical surfaces in the three areas was similar (cf. table 4), API and BRI values varied significantly between the three cemeteries (Table 6). These differences are possibly related to re-use of the burial areas at different periods. The construction of the Late Medieval cemetery next to the Early Medieval cemetery damaged both funerary structures and the human remains. Similarly, the revival of the site during the Modern Period caused damage to the Late Medieval site (Bello 2001).

Table 6: Statistically significant differences in frequency of well preserved bones and BRI values in the three areas at St. Maximin.

Differences in the frequencies of well preserved bones (API)

Modern / Early Medieval cemetery	$\chi^2 = 17.523$	p < 0.0001
Modern / Late Medieval cemetery	$\chi^2 = 18.534$	p < 0.0001

Differences in BRI values

Modern/ Early Medieval cemetery	$\chi^2 = 7.834$	p = 0.0005
Modern / Late Medieval cemetery	$\chi^2 = 11.812$	p < 0.0001

The sample from St. Estève le Pont shows the poorest preservation of cortical surfaces (cf. table 4). The differences in the state of preservation of cortical surfaces are statistically significant between St. Estève le Pont and St. Maximin ($\chi^2 = 36.52$, p< 0.0001), St. Estève le Pont and Observance ($\chi^2 = 32.07$, p< 0.0001) and St. Estève le Pont and Spitalfields ($\chi^2 = 19.422$, p< 0.0001). The agricultural exploitation of the area above the cemetery over the last 200 years caused the main alterations to the remains (Genot, 2000). The roots of plants growing above the osteological material caused both physical and chemical degradation. The roots creep into the bones and exert a strong pressure on the bone walls, causing progressive chipping and fragmentation. At the same time, they cause the dissolution of the mineral component of the bones by excreting humic acids. This "root etching" (Lyman 1996) results in progressive erosion of the cortical surface and may lead to complete dissolution of the bone. The bones of St. Estève le Pont sample exhibit wavy dendritic marks made by roots, and this erosive process caused partial dissolution of the cortical surfaces, often resulting in marked grooves and bone perforation. This type of damage can be observed in remains from all areas of this site (Bello 2001).

1.2 Grave/container characteristics

At St. Estève le Pont cemetery, subadult graves were generally shallower (depth ranging from 0.1 to 0.31 metres) than adult graves (depth ranging from 0.1 to 0.39 metres; table 7). This difference is statistically significant (t-value = -3.498, p = 0.0018). The correlation between the age of all individuals buried and the depth of their graves is also significant (for 63 degrees of freedom, Pearson R = 0.400, 1-p = 0.000473). These results suggest that the site of St. Estève Le Pont had two main patterns of funerary structures: deeper graves for adults and more superficial pits for subadults. There was no apparent relationship between the depth of adult graves and the adults' sex, although female graves were generally shallower than male graves.

Table 7: Average depth of the grave, frequencies of Well-preserved skeletons, Well Represented skeletons and Skeletons with Well Preserved Cortical Surfaces at St. Estève le Pont sample.

	Grave depth	Well Preserved	Well Represented	Preserved Surfaces
Subadult	0.21 m	15.6%	46.9%	37.5%
Adult	0.27 m	67.3%	96.2%	78.8%

The correlation between grave depth and the preservation of the individuals buried (e.g. frequency of well preserved skeletons) was highly significant (for 63 degrees of freedom, Pearson R = 0.327, 1-p = 0.003892).

Table 8: Frequencies of Well Preserved Skeletons, Well Represented Skeletons and Skeletons with Well Preserved Cortical Surfaces for the individuals buried inside and outside coffins, Named sample and Un-coffined sample (Spitalfields).

| | inside coffin | | | outside coffin | |
	Subadults	Adults	total	Adults	total
No individuals	87	282	369	20	21
Well Preserved Skeletons	51.2%	74.5%	68.4%	70.0%	66.7%
Well Represented Skeletons	64.4%	87.2%	82.3%	75.0%	76.2%
Skeletons Well Preserved Cortical Surfaces	88.5%	96.1%	94.8%	95.0%	95.2%

The correlation between grave depth and bone representation for the individuals buried (frequency of well represented skeletons) was also highly significant (for 63 degrees of freedom, Pearson R = 0.334, 1-p = 0.003273). Conversely, there was no correlation between grave depth and the state of preservation of the cortical surface of the bones. These results suggest that grave depth can influence both preservation and representation of osseous remains (the deeper the grave, the better preserved and more abundant the bones), but it does not influence the state of preservation of cortical surfaces. Nevertheless, if the hypothesis that the deeper the grave, the better preserved and the more abundant the bones is true, we should find a uniform state of preservation if all remains were buried at the same depth. At Observance site, the individuals were all buried in the same grave and under the same burial conditions. In this sample, subadult bones are generally less well preserved and less abundant than adult bones (cf. Table 4). The similarities in the patterns of preservation observed at St. Estève le Pont and Observance suggest that grave depth does not determine differences in the state of preservation of osseous material, contrary to Acsàdi and Nemeskéri (1970). It seems more likely that the differences in the preservation of adult and subadult remains are mainly due to anatomical features of the bones (e.g. size, shape, density), while the taphonomic characteristics of the site may have a secondary influence upon susceptibility of bone to decay.

In the Spitalfields sample, it was noted that the presence of coffins had provided better protection for the osseous remains. Remains buried without coffins were generally less well preserved and with bones less abundant than those buried inside coffins (table 8). The characteristics of the coffins themselves did not seem directly linked to specific preservation patterns (table 9). In particular, the coffins observed in the Spitalfields crypt were made with one, two or three shells. The coffins with three shells seemed to provide better protection from taphonomic agents than those with one or two shells but these differences were not statistically significant. The coffin shells were made of wood only, lead only or both wood

and lead. Most individuals were buried in coffins made of wood and lead. No subadults were buried in coffins made of lead only, but the number of subadults and adults buried in coffins made of wood only or of both wood and lead was similar. None of the differences in the state of preservation based on the coffin construction material was statistically significant.

Table 9: Frequencies of skeletons with well preserved, well represented and Well Preserved Cortical Surfaces, by coffin type, Named sample (Spitalfields).

Coffin Type[1]		Sub adult	Adult	Total
	% individuals	*32.9*	*19.0*	**22.1**
01	*% Well-Preserved*	*45.2*	*62.0*	**56.5**
	% Well-Represented	*71.0*	*81.5*	**77.6**
	% Well Preserved Surfaces	*93.5*	*94.4*	**94.1**
	% individuals	*2.4*	*11.6*	**9.6**
03	*% Well-Preserved*	*50.0*	*60.6*	**60.0**
	% of Well-Represented	*50.0*	*69.7*	**68.6**
	% Well Preserved Surfaces	*100*	*93.9*	**94.3**
	% individuals	*8.5*	*3.2*	**4.4**
36	*% Well-Preserved*	*57.2*	*44.4*	**50.0**
	% Well-Represented	*71.4*	*66.7*	**68.8**
	% Well Preserved Surfaces	*85.7*	*66.7*	**75.0**
	% individuals	*14.6*	*30.1*	**30.1**
38	*% Well-Preserved*	*41.7*	*80.6*	**76.4**
	% Well-Represented	*58.3*	*92.9*	**89.1**
	% Well Preserved Surfaces	*93.3*	*94.9*	**93.6**
	% individuals	*39.0*	*23.2*	**26.8**
66	*% Well-Preserved*	*50.0*	*84.8*	**73.5**
	% Well-Represented	*78.1*	*98.5*	**91.8**
	% Well Preserved Surfaces	*87.5*	*100*	**95.9**

[1]Type *01*: 1 shell, wood outer; *type 03*: 2 shell, wood outer and wood inner ; *type 36*: 2 shell, wood outer, lead inner ; *type 38*: 3 shell: wood outer, lead inner, wood inner, lid; *type 66*: 3 shell: wood outer, lead inner, wood outer, lid (according to Reeve and Adams, 1993)

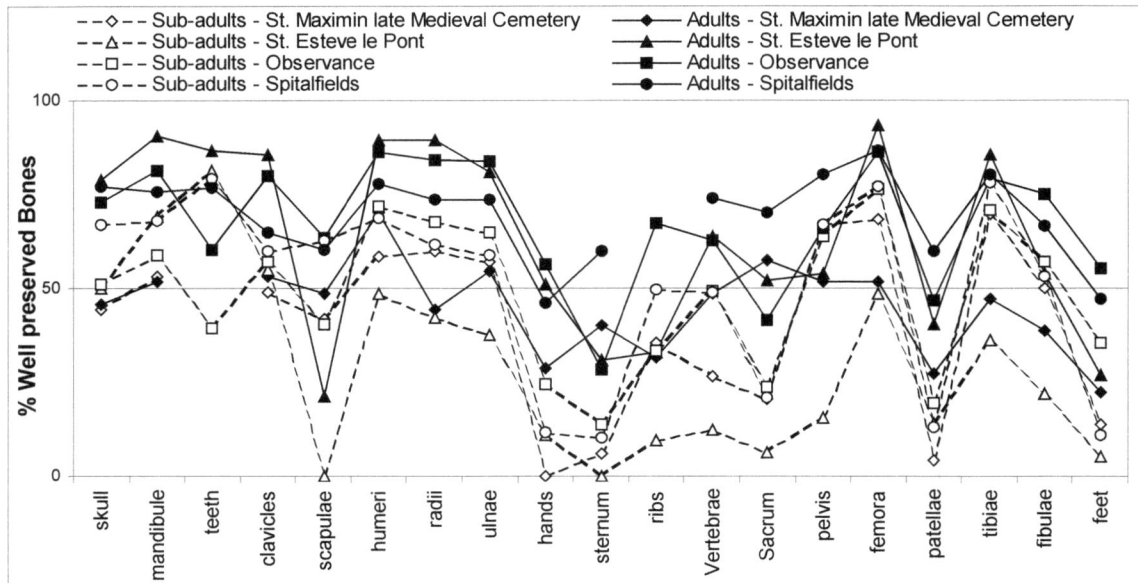

Figure 1: Frequencies of Well Preserved Bones in the four samples observed.

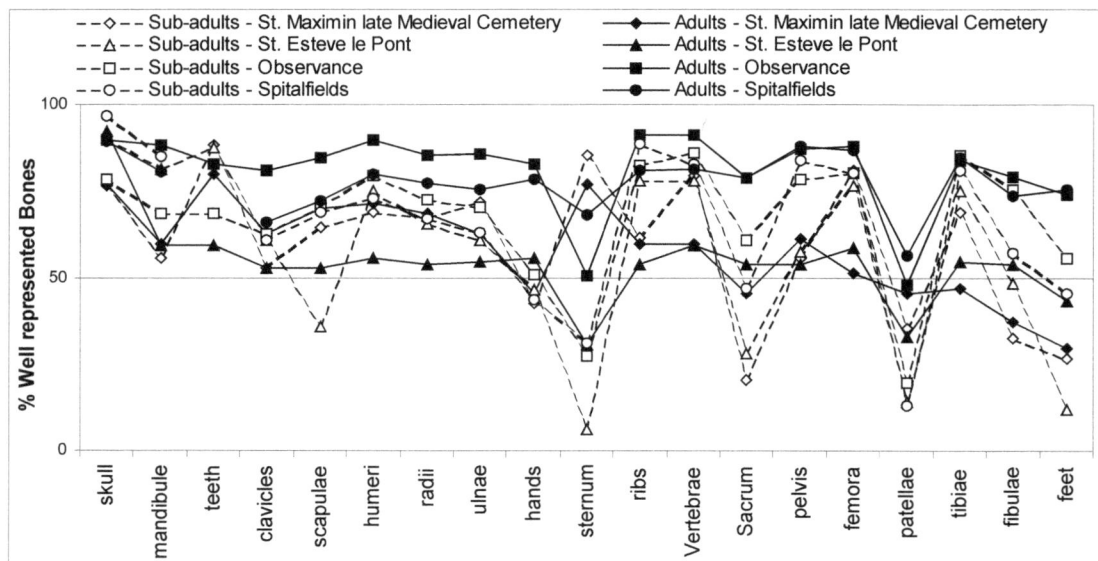

Figure 2: Frequencies of Well Represented Bones in the four samples observed.

2 Intrinsic factors

Frequencies of well preserved and well represented bones were estimated for both adult and subadult individuals in the four studied collections. The representation of the frequencies of well preserved and well represented bones by curbs has no mathematical significant, it only allows a better visual comprehension. In the case of St. Maximin, only the Late Medieval cemetery was taken into account in order to avoid the combination of remains with different taphonomic histories (Fig. 1 and 2).

In all four samples, scapulae, sterna, vertebrae, sacra, patellae and hand and foot bones showed the lowest frequencies of well preserved bones.

The scapula was generally poorly preserved because of the fragility of the sub-scapular fossa. Nevertheless, with the exception of subadult scapulae in the St. Estève le Pont sample, representation of this bone was generally higher than 50% and comparable to that of the clavicle. This relative abundance of scapulae was mainly due to the good preservation of the acromion spine, the coracoid process and the lateral border by of the infraglenoid tubercle, all of which have high bone density.

Vertebral columns were generally abundant (we considered a vertebral column present when at least one vertebra or a fragment of a vertebra was present). In the St. Maximin and St. Estève le Pont samples lumbar vertebrae had the highest WPB frequencies, while for the Observance sample, cervical vertebrae had the highest frequencies and for Spitalfields the thoracic vertebrae. The good preservation of lumbar vertebrae is probably associated with their shape and structural robusticity, while the good preservation of cervical vertebrae, especially C1 and C2, could be due to the protection afforded by the skull when the skeleton is articulated.

The sacrum, like vertebral bodies, is characterised by low bone density and a high proportion of cancellous bone (Boaz & Behrensmeyer 1976; Münzel 1988). Accordingly, it was often fragmented and poorly preserved in all the observed collections. On all samples, it was observed that the portions most resistant to taphonomic processes were the median sacral crest and the promontory of the first sacral vertebra.

Ribs fragments are generally abundant in osteoarchaeological samples, but their anatomical identification can be difficult limiting their use in MNI calculations (Bello 2001).

The sternum was often fragmented, again due to low bone density. The manubrium was the best preserved and most abundant portion, as seen at other sites (Brézillon 1963; Waldron 1987).

The small bones of the hands and feet are generally poorly represented in osteoarchaeological collections, but tend to be well preserved and almost complete when present (Bello et al. 2003). The good preservation of hand and foot bones has been ascribed to the reduction of the medullary cavity (Guthrie 1967), facilitating complete preservation of these bones even in very fragmented and damaged collections (Defleur et al. 1993). In the observed samples, hand bones were more abundant than foot bones (we considered a hand/foot present when at least one carpal/tarsal, metacarpal/metatarsal, phalange, or a fragment of one of these bones was present). Metacarpals and metatarsals were generally more abundant than carpal and tarsal bones. The frequency of phalanges, of both hands and feet, was directly related to their dimensions, with proximal phalanges being more abundant than middle phalanges, and the latter more abundant than distal phalanges (Bello et al. 2003). Nevertheless, none of these differences were statistically significant.

Patellae were under-represented in the samples studied, but tended to be almost complete when present.

The frequencies of well preserved and well represented skeletal elements in the four studied collections show great similarity:

1. subadult bones were generally less well preserved and less abundant than adult bones.

2. the less mineralised and smaller bones of the skeleton were generally less well preserved and less well represented than the denser and larger bones.

These results suggest a consistent relationship between size and survival of human anatomical remains. Experimental work (Bouchud 1977; Von Endt & Ortner 1984; Lambert et al. 1985) has shown that rates of decay are inversely proportional to bone size. It is therefore conceivable that the small size of bones would be disadvantaged in their preservation: they are more vulnerable to decay and loss during lifting at excavation. Moreover, since the relative volume of bones is related to an individual's age, it is probable that the bones of younger infants should be more affected than the bones of older subadults and adults.

Bone mineral density (BMD, defined as mass of mineral per unit of volume) decreases in the first month after birth followed by a rapid increase during the next two years of life with slower changes thereafter (Rauch & Schoenau 2001). Guy and co-authors (1997) showed that bone density and mineral content decrease after birth, maintaining a minimum value during the first year of life. Further studies should clarify the importance of bone density in determining the difference in the preservation and survivability between subadult and adult bones.

Discussion

The taphonomic analyses of these four skeletal samples suggest that intrinsic factors are the agent mainly responsible for differing preservation patterns, whereas extrinsic factors mainly augment the effects of intrinsic characteristics.

Any process determining the selective preservation of specific bones or subgroups of individuals has a direct influence on anthropological interpretations.

In osteometrical studies, any taphonomic process that results in the selective preservation of more robust bones will produce an incongruous relationship between the osteometrical profile of the sample observed and that of the more complete (original) assemblage from which it was derived (Bello 2004).

Any difference in preservation of subadult and adult individuals has an extensive impact on palaeo-demographical reconstruction and ethnological interpretation. For example, at St. Estève le Pont site, a discrepancy was found between the number of graves (87 in all, one containing the remains of a woman and her unborn child) and the skeletal sample (84 individuals), four graves being empty. The presence of shells of gastropods (*Cecicula Ceciloides*, a 3-4 mm long gastropod whose ecology is associated with a rapid inhumation of dead bodies; Dedet et al., 1991) in these four empty pits suggested that they had probably contained bodies whose bones were not preserved. It may be assumed that the length of the pit was proportional to the height of the individual buried and that this would be linked to the subject's age. The four empty tombs were respectively 41 cm, 72 cm, 82 cm and 88 cm long. The average length of the tombs for infants aged between 0 and 2 years was 94 cm, and 99 cm for children aged 3-4 years old. These values suggest that the empty tombs most likely contained infants aged less than 2 years, whose remains had not been preserved (Bello et al. accepted paper b). This hypothesis of non-preservation of very young subadult remains was sustained by the observation that, in all samples studied, subadults' bones were generally less well preserved and less abundant than adult bones. Nevertheless, although the presence of burial structures at the St. Estève le Pont site facilitated palaeodemographical reconstruction, such interpretations cannot be made in the case of multiple and collective burials where individual graves cannot be discerned.

This evidence not only has palaeodemographical repercussions, but also social and ethnographical implications. Differences in the treatment of a body according to its social and/or biological status can indicate the egalitarian or selective nature of the living population. If the absence of a subgroup of people in a grave is interpreted purely as the result of a cultural practice, without considering the impact of intrinsic factors upon the preservation of the remains, the funerary behaviour of the population may be misunderstood.

Finally, the representation of bones, the degree of fragmentation and the preservation of cortical surfaces, all play an important role in palaeopathological and palaeoepidemiological diagnoses. The absence of hand and foot bones, of patellae and thoracic vertebrae can lead to the over-estimation of the prevalence of degenerative disease (Bello 2001). Peri-mortem traumatic lesions can be misinterpreted as a fragmentation process, resulting in an under-estimation of traumatic prevalence. The preservation of cortical surfaces directly influences the interpretation of pathological infectious anomalies. On the one hand, the taphonomic processes may be interpreted as pathological alterations; while on the other hand, damaged cortical surfaces do not allow exhaustive diagnosis. In the case of the St. Estève le Pont sample, for example, the pronounced alteration of cortical surfaces resulted in an under-estimation of infectious disease, and thereby limited all palaeoepidemiological comparisons with contemporary sites (Bello et al. in press).

Conclusion

The inclusion of burial practices and burial structures under taphonomic processes will define a new taphonomic model, which may give the word taphonomy a wider meaning. In these terms, taphonomy describes all natural and cultural processes leading to damage of bones, from the death of the individual to the final laboratory analysis.

The impact of all these taphonomic processes on the state of preservation of human remains must be mitigated by the intrinsic characteristics of the bones, as the state of preservation and representation of osseous remains seems mainly dependent on the size and density of bones themselves. Strong taphonomic processes can nevertheless increase intrinsic susceptibilities of bones to decay.

The impact of taphonomic processes, burial practices and anatomical bone features on the state of preservation of osteoarchaeological samples needs to be considered in order to minimise the risk of bias in any anthropological (both biological and ethnological) interpretation of past populations.

Literature cited

Acsàdi G and Nemeskéri J (1970) *History of Human Life Span and Mortality.* Budapest: Akadémiai Kiadó.

Bello S (2001) *Taphonomie des restes osseux humains. Effet des processus de conservation du squelette sur les paramètres anthropologiques.* Marseilles: Università degli Studi di Firenze, Florence, Italy and Université de la Méditerranée. Unpublished PhD.

Bello S, Signoli M, Rabino-Massa E, and Dutour O (2002) Les processus de conservation différentielle du squelette des individus immatures. Implications sur les reconstitutions paléodémographiques. *Bulletins et Mémoires de la Société d'Anthropologie de Paris* 14 (3-4): 245-262.

Bello S, Thomann A, Lalys L, Signoli M, Rabino-Massa E, and Dutour O (2003) Calcul du "Profil théorique de survie osseuse la plus probable" et son utilisation dans l'interprétation des processus taphonomiques pouvant déterminer la formation d'un échantillon ostéologique humain. British Archaeological Reports, International Series 1145. Oxford: BAR Publishing; 21-30

Bello S (2004) Taphonomy, selective preservation and robusticity in human skeletal samples: the osteometric paradox. *American Journal of Physical Anthropology*, suppl. 38: 61-62.

Bello S, Signoli M, Thomann A, Lalys L, and Dutour O (in press) Nouvelle méthode de quantification de l'état de conservation des surfaces corticales et son application dans les études paléopathologiques et paléoépidémiologiques. *Bulletins et Mémoires de la Société d'Anthropologie de Paris* 15.

Bello S and Andrews P. (accepted paper a) How can the state of preservation of human bones increase the understanding of funerary practices? In C Knusel and R Gowland (eds.): *The Social Archaeology of Funerary Remains.* Oxford: Oxbow Books.

Bello S, Thomann A, Signoli M, Dutour O, and Andrews P (accepted paper b) Age and sex bias in the reconstruction of past populations' structures. *American Journal of Physical Anthropology.*

Birkner R (1980) *L'image radiologique typique du squelette.* Paris: Maloine.

Boaz NT and Behrensmeyer AK (1976) Hominid taphonomy: transport of Human skeletal parts in an Artificial Fluviatile Environment. *American Journal of Physical Anthropology* 45 (1): 53-60.

Bouchud J (1977) Etude de la conservation différentielle des os des dents. *Bulletin de l'Association Française pour l'Etude du Quaternaire Supplément* 47: 69-73.

Brézillon M (1963) L'Hypogée des Mournouards. Démographie. *Gallia Préhistorica* V (1): 50-63.

Builkstra JE and Ubelaker DH (1994) *Standards for Data Collection from Human Skeletal Remains.* Fayetteville, Arkansas: Arkansas Archeological Survey Research, series n. 44.

Dedet B, Duday H, and Tillier AM (1991) Inhumation de fœtus, nouveau-nés et nourrissons dans les habitats protohistoriques du Languedoc: l'exemple de Gailhan (Gard). *Gallia* 48: 59-108.

Defleur A, Dutour O, and Valladas H (1993) Cannibals among the Neanderthals? *Nature* 362: 214.

Dodson P and Wexlar D (1979) Taphonomic investigations of owl pellets. *Paleobiology* 5: 279-284.

Fazekas IG and Kosa F (1978) *Forensic fetal osteology.* Budapest: Akadémiai Kiado.

Genot A (2000) *Saint-Estève-le-Pont, Opérations II et III. D.F.S. de fouille nécessitée par l'urgence absolue (21 juin –16 juillet 1999) et fouille d'évaluation archéologique (06 – 10 septembre 1999).* Université de la Méditerranée: Marseilles. Unpublished Report.

Genovés S (1959) L'estimation des différences sexuelles dans l'os coxal: differences métriques et différences morphologiques. *Bulletins et Mémoires de la Société D'Anthropologie de Paris* 10: 3-95.

Guthrie RD (1967) Differential preservation and recovery of Pleistocene large mammal remains in Alaske. *Journal of Paleontology* 41: 243-246.

Guy H, Masset C, and Baud CA (1997) Infant taphonomy. *International Journal of Osteoarchaeology* 7: 221-229.

Henderson J (1987) Factors determining the state of preservation of human remains. In A Boddington, AN Garland and RC Janaway (eds.) *Approaches to archaeology and forensic science.* Manchester: Manchester University Press; 43-54.

Hoyme LES (1984) Sex differenciation in the posterior pelvis. *Coll. Anthrop.* 8: 139-153.

Iscan MY (1989) *Age markers in the human skeleton.* Springfield: Charles C. Thomas.

Lamandin H (1978) Critère dentaire pour appréciation d'âge: étude de la translucidité et des canalicules, intérêt en odontostomatologie légale. *Revue d'Odonto-Stomatologie* VII (2): 11-119.

Lambert JB, Simpson SV, Weiner JG, and Buikstra JE (1985) Induced metal-iron exchange in excavated human bone. *Journal of Archaeological Science* 12: 85-92.

Lyman RL (1996) *Vertebrate taphonomy.* Cambridge: Cambridge University Press.

Margerison BJ and Knüsel CJ (2002) A comparison of attritional and catastrophic cemeteries: the palaeo-demography of the Medieval Plague cemetery at the Mint Site, London. *American Journal of Physical Anthropology* 119(2): 134-143.

Miles AEW (1963) The dentition in the assessment of individual age in skeletal material. In DR Brothwell (ed.): *Dental Anthropology.* London: Pergamon Press; 191-209.

Molleson T and Cox M (1993) T*he Spitalfields Project. Volume 2 – The Anthropology. The Middling Sort.* CBA Research Report 86. York: Council for British Archaeology.

Münzel SC (1988) Quantitative analysis and archaeological site interpretation. *Archaeozoologia* II (1, 2): 93-110.

Perrin F (2000) Le mort et la mort en Gaule à l'âge du fer (VIIIe-Ier S. av.J.-C.), In E Crubézy, C Masset, E Lorans, F Perrin, and L Tranoy (eds.): *Archéologie funéraire* Paris: Edition Errance; 86-102.

Rauch F and Schoenau E (2001) Changes in bone density during childhood and adolescence: An approach based on bone's biological organization. *Journal of Bone and Mineral Research* 90 (4): 597-604.

Reeve J and Adams M (1993) *The Spitalfields Project. Volume 1 – The Archaeology. Across the STYX.* CBA Research Report 85. York: Council for British Archaeology.

Scheuer L and Black S (2000) *Developmental Juvenile Osteology.* San Diego (CA): Academic Press.

Stewart TD (1957) The rate of development of vertebral hypertrophic arthritis and its utility in age estimation. *American Journal of Physical Anthropology* 15: 433.

Stewart TD (1979) *Essentials of forensic anthropology.* Springfield: Charles C Thomas.

Tranoy L (2000) La mort en Gaule romaine. In Crubézy E, Masset C, Lorans E, Perrin F and Tranoy L. (eds.) *Archéologie funéraire.* Paris: Edition Errance; 105-153.

Ubelaker DH (1989). *Human skeletal remains: excavation, analysis and interpretation.* 2nd edn. Smithsonian Institution, Manuals on Archaeology 2. Washington: Taraxum.

Von Endt DW and Ortner DJ (1984) Experimental effects of bone size and temperature on bone diagenesis. *Journal of Archaeological Sciences* 11: 247-253.

Waldron T (1987) The relative survival of the human skeleton: implications for palaeopathology. In A Boddington, AN Garland, and RC Janaway. (eds.): *Death, decay and reconstruction.* Manchester: Manchester University Press; 55-64

White DT and Folkens PA (1991) *Human Osteology.* London: Academic Press.

Peri- and post mortem surface features on archaeological human bone: why they should not be ignored and a protocol for their identification and interpretation.

Peri- and post-mortem surface features

Louise Loe & Margaret Cox

Forensic and Bioarchaeological Sciences Group
School of Conservation Sciences
Talbot Campus
Bournemouth University
Poole, Dorset, BH12 5BB.
* e-mail address for correspondence: lloe@bournemouth.ac.uk
Tel.: +44 (0) 1202 595661; Fax: +44 (0) 1202 595255

Abstract

This paper focuses on peri- and post-mortem surface features, or modifications that alter the surface of the bone around the time of death and after death until examination in the laboratory. A protocol for recording these features is presented and some of the limitations associated with their identification and interpretation discussed. An example from Fishmonger Swallet, Alveston, Gloucestershire is presented to highlight why and how surface features should be an integral part of any study that explores fracture morphologies and fragmentation patterns in archaeological human bone assemblages.

Key words: peri- and post-mortem modification; anthropogenic alterations; taphonomy

Introduction

Surface features are alterations to the cortex of bone that are the result of human (e.g. tool marks), faunal (e.g. gnawing) and environmental (e.g. sediment abrasion) activity. These may occur on the sub-periosteal surface of the bone, penetrate the bony cortex, or penetrate the medullary cavity of long bones and the endocranial surface of the skull. Surface features are an integral part of modification analysis; they aid the interpretation of fracture morphologies and fragmentation patterns within and between assemblages that may be the result of many factors including deliberate breakage, trampling, sediment pressure, weathering and excavation and post-excavation damage. This paper discusses a method employed in a wider study exploring peri- and post-mortem modification in human bone collections curated in the United Kingdom. The importance of surface features in reconstructing the events surrounding death and burial in the past is demonstrated. In particular, it is stressed that, in order to understand fracture morphologies and fragmentation patterns, interpretation is not possible without scoring the presence or absence of these and, when present, examining in detail their morphology at both a macroscopic and microscopic level. This is demonstrated with an example from Fishmonger Swallet.

Present Study of Surface Features

Recent work (Cox 2001; O'Sullivan 2001; Schulting & Wysocki 2002; Smith & Brickley 2004; Wysocki & Whittle 2000), which has identified evidence for anthropogenic alterations, has highlighted the fact that the analysis of this and other aspects of peri- and post-mortem modification are neglected areas in anthropology in the U.K. This largely concerns prehistoric collections excavated at a time when interest tended to focus on palaeopathology and the assessment of morphological and metrical traits.

Exceptions include work by Cook (1986) on possible cut marks on a prehistoric skull from Gough's cave, and studies of cut marks found on Roman neonatal bones from Poundbury Camp (Molleson & Cox 1988) and on a prehistoric mandible from Millin Bay, Co. Down (Murphy 2003). There are several published reports on cranial tool marks such as trepanation (McKinley 1992; Roberts and McKinley 2003; Wells 1974, Parry 1952), scalping and defleshing (Mays and Steele 1996), decapitation (Boylston et al. 2000; Harman et al. 1981) and sharp weapon injuries (Novak 2000; Wells 1981). Cut marks to the skull as the result of edged weapons have, in particular, received the most attention in the literature to date (Anderson 1996; Boylston et al. 2000; Novak 2000). However, very few papers focus on modifications affecting the post-cranial skeleton.

Table 1. The main characteristic features to score when recording striations

Trait	Feature
Location	Zone & aspect (anterior/ posterior/ superior/ inferior/ medial/ lateral)
Frequency	Multiple/ single
Concentration	Isolated/ clustered/ disparate
Orientation	Parallel to the long axis of the bone/ transverse to the long axis of the bone.
Direction of multiple striations	Uni-directional/ multi-directional
Travelling direction	Indeterminate/ superior right – inferior left/ superior – inferior/ medial - lateral, etc.
Margin texture	Rough/ smooth/ sharp/ abraded/ jagged/ polished/ flaked
Margin appearance in plan	Straight/ curved/ irregular
Relationship of striations	Parallel/ sub-parallel/ non-parallel/ criss-cross/ clustered/ disparate
Shape in profile	'v'- shaped /, 'u'-shaped, 'w'-shaped, other (e.g. square 'u' shape) & Deep/ narrow/ sharp/ blunt
Depth	Follows the contour of the bone/ cuts into the surface of the bone. If cuts into the surface: Cuts the cortical surface/ penetrates medullary or endocranial surface
Internal wall texture (score each separately)	Rough/ smooth/ sharp/ abraded/ jagged/ polished/ flaked
Internal wall appearance (score each separately)	Straight/ concave/ stepped/ irregular & Steep/ gradual/ indeterminate & Microstriations/ crushing / indeterminate
Colour of exposed surface	Clean/ soiled/ same colour as the surrounding bone

(based on Blumenschine et al. 1996; Blumenschine & Selvaggio 1988; Greenfield 2000; Haglund et al. 1988; O'Sullivan 2001; Shipman & Rose 1983; Shipman 1981).

Much of our knowledge relating to peri- and post-mortem surface features derives from anecdotal evidence. In Britain, there are few studies that focus on bone modification to be found in the literature As a result, the extent and range of peri- and post-mortem surface features in human skeletal collections that are curated in this country is largely unknown.

Future Study of Surface Features

It is important that surface features analysis moves beyond the case study approach, as has successfully been achieved in trauma analysis. Analysis needs to be undertaken on large samples to examine within and between assemblage patterns, as well as temporal and spatial trends (Lovejoy & Heiple 1981). In this way social, cultural and environmental factors can be explored. Before this may be attempted, however, methods for recording and interpreting surface features need to be developed and advanced.

Most current methods derive from American studies, but the extent to which these apply to material derived from a British archaeological context is questionable. For example, detailed studies (e.g. Binford 1981; Blumenschine 1988; Brain 1981; Sutcliff 1973) of faunal scavenging activities are biased towards carnivores (especially hyenas, leopards and dogs) but these account for only a fraction, if any, of the species that would have been native to ancient Britain, if at all. Less attention has been given to the scavenging activities of rodents and antydactyls (Brothwell 1976; Haglund et al. 1988; Sutcliff 1973), least of all to non-mammalian animals

such as crabs, fish and birds, despite being known to scavenge human remains (Haglund et al. 1988).

Research also needs to focus on specific British burial environments, such as swallets and barrows, and to explore the different taphonomic processes and agents in these contexts that may alter bone surfaces. Attention needs to be given to those processes and agents that may mimic genuine cut marks or other anthropogenic modifications. Although discussion exists in the literature on pseudo cut marks as the result of trampling and sediment abrasion (Behrensmeyer et al. 1986; Haynes 1986; Olsen & Shipman 1988), this can only be applied in a very broad sense.

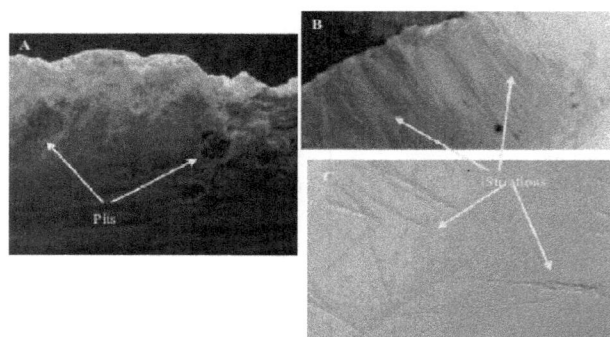

Figure 1. Experimentally produced pits and striations resulting from carnivore gnawing (a), rodent gnawing (b), and defleshing (c). *(Specimen (a) prepared by I. O'Sullivan, specimen (b) prepared by N.Bryant and specimen (c) prepared by P. Harding; photographs by L.Loe).*

More generally, minimum criteria for identifying, recording and interpreting surface features are yet to be fully explored. For example, it is unclear how much detailed investigation - whether macroscopic or microscopic - is required in order accurately to identify and interpret surface features, and the extent to which this may vary at inter- and intra-observer levels (Blumenschine et al, 1996). Techniques for osteologists, who work in a contract environment and do not have the time for detailed investigation, also need to be addressed.

A Protocol for Recording Surface Features

Surface features may be broadly classified as pits and striations (Fig. 1) as these are the most frequently observed bone alterations modified by human, animal and environmental agencies (Shipman 1981). Criteria for their identification are described in detail elsewhere (e.g. Blumenschine et al. 1996; Blumenschine & Selvaggio 1988; O'Sullivan 2001; Shipman & Rose 1983; Shipman 1981) and are summarised in Tables 1 and 2.

Table 2. The main characteristic features to score when recording pits

Trait	Feature
Location	Zone and aspect (anterior/ posterior/ superior/ inferior/ medial/ lateral)
Frequency	Multiple/ single
Concentration	Isolated/ clustered/ disparate
Shape in profile	Bowl – shaped, 'U'-shaped, other
Depth	Deep/shallow
Internal wall appearance (score each separately)	Straight/ concave/ stepped/ irregular & Steep/ gradual/ indeterminate & Microstriations/ crushing / indeterminate
Internal wall texture (score each separately)	Rough/ smooth/ sharp/ abraded/ jagged/ polished/ flaked
Apex	Present/ absent/ indeterminate & Well defined/ indistinct
Margin texture	Rough/ smooth/ sharp/ abraded/ jagged/ polished/ flaked
Margin appearance in plan	Circular/ sub-circular/ semi-circular
Colour of exposed surface	Clean/ same colour as the surrounding bone

(based on Blumenschine et al., 1996; Blumenschine & Selvaggio 1988; Greenfield 2000; Haglund et al. 1988; O'Sullivan 2001; Shipman & Rose 1983; Shipman 1981).

Methods employed to study surface features derive from the forensic and zooarchaeological literature. These primarily aim to identify the following:

1. The agent (e.g. human, animal, or environmental cause),

2. Timing (e.g. features will display characteristic changes depending on whether they occurred when the bone was fresh (i.e. the protein had survived), or mineralised (i.e. the protein had decayed)),

3. The actor (e.g. human or animal) and the effector (e.g. tool or tooth).

A detailed protocol that scores characteristics qualitatively and quantitatively should be employed to diagnose these. Examination should be undertaken under a bright artificial light with a 10x hand lens. All elements should be inspected by slowly rotating them relative to the light source (Blumenschine et al. 1996). The level to which macroscopic analysis should be undertaken is a matter of continued debate and requires further research (see below). In the interim, a light stereo microscope with a range of magnifications is recommended for scanning surfaces, as well as scanning electron microscopy to identify features that cannot otherwise be identified. The degree to which elements are scanned microscopically will vary depending upon the research objectives and the assemblage being examined.

Quantitative analysis needs to focus not only on measuring the length, width and when appropriate the depth of a feature, but also on the relationship of that feature to other modifications that might be present (O'Sullivan 2001). Identifying the relationship between modifications on the same element may enable a clearer picture of the type of event responsible for the modifications observed. For example, pits and grooves that lie within 5mm of a peri-mortem fracture margin are interpreted as the result of percussion activity with a hammerstone and anvil (Blumenschine & Selvaggio 1988).

Qualitative analysis involves recording factors such as the location, orientation, frequency, concentration, direction, profile, texture, plan, internal appearance and colour of features (Tables 1 and 2). These are described in more detail elsewhere (Blumenschine &Selvaggio 1988; Hurlburt 2000; O'Sullivan 2001; Shipman 1981).

The importance of describing the anatomical distribution of surface features is widely recognised (Blumenschine & Selvaggio 1988, 1991; Blumenschine et al. 1996) but methods employed to do this have received less attention, the general procedure being to record location in terms of the proximal, middle or distal portions of the bone (Buikstra & Ubeklaker 1994). However, as with fracture patterns (Knüsel & Outram 2004), this hinders the interpretation of surface features as it does not record their relationship to areas of muscle attachment and other anatomical landmarks, which hold significant implications for their interpretation. Striations caused by cut marks as a result of disarticulation and defleshing tend to occur in the region of muscle attachments and around joints (Hurlburt 2000), whereas striations caused by animal gnawing tend to occur on prominent surfaces of bones (Buikstra & Ubelaker 1994). To this end, location should be recorded with reference to the anatomical zone in which the feature occurs (Knüsel & Outram 2004) in addition to its location within a zone (e.g. antero-medial /antero-lateral, postero-medial/postero-lateral and proximal, middle or distal portions of the zone).

Based on these qualitative and quantitative observations, features may be classified according to the most likely actor and effector using the criteria described in Table 3. Not all features will fulfil every criterion as there is enormous cross over between categories, and no features are exclusive to a particular agent. The use of stone tools for example may cause some surface features that might reflect nothing more than the simple interaction between stone and bone (Cook 1986: 284; Oliver 1989: 91). Marks made by stone on bone may result from mechanically identical movements and yet be related to quite different events (e.g. a human drawing a stone as a tool across bone or a sharp stone being drawn across bone in the context of trampling). It is recommended, therefore, that differential diagnoses of actor and effector are employed and particular attention is given to the broader contextual factors listed in Table 3.

Some Limitations

Determining timing after mineralisation but before recovery

An alteration may be determined peri-mortem if the bony response is typical of fresh (i.e. bone that has an intact organic matrix) bone, or post-mortem if the response is typical of mineralised bone (Wakely 1997). While it is relatively straightforward to identify post-mortem features that have occurred on mineralised bone as a result of excavation and recovery, it is much harder to distinguish features that occur prior to excavation and recovery, but after the bone has mineralised (O'Sullivan 2001). Attention to location and other associated features are therefore essential in order to address this problem.

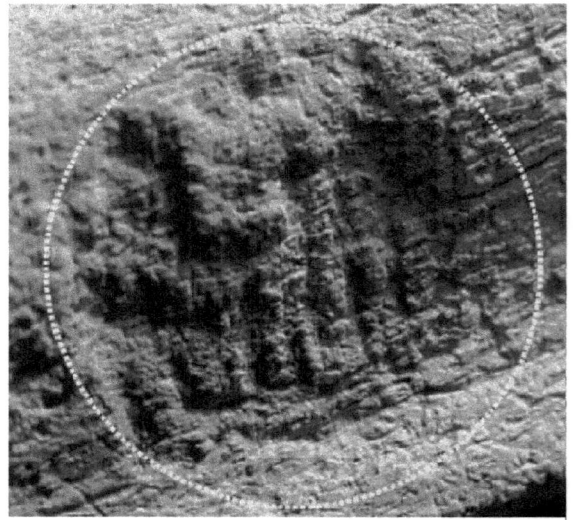

Figure 2. Illustration of how abrasion can limit the interpretation of surface features. The circled area shows what appears to be a dense patch of unidirectional sub-parallel striations, suggestive of percussion marks. However, abrasion obscures their morphology, hindering interpretation. *(Photographed by L.Loe).*

Obscured features

Features may, over time, become abraded and lose their defining characteristics. Although experimental work has shown that slicing marks can appear flatter and wider after being abraded (Shipman and Rose 1983:80), the effects of abrasion on other features (e.g. percussion striations; Fig. 2) are yet to be explored. Also lacking is knowledge of the limitations imposed on interpretation when a bone has been modified to the extent that 'earlier' modifications have been obscured. For example, if a fracture margin has been scavenged, any evidence that may suggest what had caused the fracture (e.g. associated percussion abrasions as a result of breaking open the bone with a hammer-stone) may be obscured. This 'taphonomic overprinting' (Shipman & Rose 1983: 60) means that in order to interpret these cases, fractures must be analysed at the assemblage level and not in isolation. In this sense then, surface features can also hinder analyses of fracture morphologies and fragmentation.

Table 3. Criteria for identifying actor and effector

Actor	Effector	Feature	Characteristic features — Metal tool	Characteristic features — Stone tool	Context
Human	Metal or stone tool	Cut/slice marks	Deep steep sided regular elongate groove; 'v'- or hard cornered 'u'-shaped cross-section; well defined apex; sometimes have internal longitudinal micro-striations of uniform depth and spacing; clean internal appearance[1].	Shallow wide irregular groove with uneven 'v'-shaped cross section; indistinct apex; walls tend to be concave rather than straight; one relatively steep, smooth wall and one gradual rough wall; internal parallel longitudinal micro-striations of uneven length and thickness which tend to occur on one wall more than the other ('shoulder effects'); micro-striations may give the impression of a series of shallow interconnected grooves; sometimes have small hooks ('barbs') at either end[2].	Anatomically meaningful locations (i.e. near articulations or in areas of muscle, tendon and ligament attachment)[3]; Have a function or purpose[4]; the distribution of cut/chop/scrape marks shows symmetry and repetitive patterning within the individual and the sample; absence of factors in the burial environment that could potentially mimic metal or flint marks (cut, scrape or chop)[5]; clustered rather than isolated; evidence of repeated interaction with the same sharp edge[6].
Human	Metal or stone tool	Cut/slice marks	**Metal and stone tool** — Single elongate groove; no internal crushing; cut into surface of the bone; tend to be transverse to long axis; often occur in sub-parallel groups.		As above
		Chop marks	Usually transverse to long axis; elongate groove; contain internal crushing; lack internal parallel striations; compared to cut and scrape marks, broader top in profile and shorter in plan[7].		
		Scrape marks	Multiple fine striations; occur in broad shallow fields; not confined to a single main groove; Shallow 'v'-shaped cross-section; often parallel to long axis[8].		
Human	Hammerstone and anvil	Percussion marks	Occur in dense superficial patches; orientated transverse to the long axis of the bone; observe a strict uni-directionality; are straight and parallel; have shallow 'v'-shaped cross sections; less well defined than cut marks; often occur within or flank a percussion groove; often emanate from or are within percussion pits; grooves and pits lack crushing[9].		Associated flake scars; concentrated in areas of marrow exposure; within 5mm of peri-mortem fracture margin[10], usually confined to cortex; often at or opposite point of percussion impact[11]; common on large mid-shaft fragments and/or notched fragments and flakes[12].

15

Table 3: continued

Environmental	Sediment	Scratch /score	Multi-directional; often faint; shallow, 'v'- , 'u'- or 'w'-shaped cross-section; uneven thickness and depth; tend to cross, intersect, and curve; tend to lack fine parallel, internal microstriations; may be isolated or occur as a group[13].	Absence of obvious patterning and location; tends not to respect areas of muscle, tendon and ligament attachment; tends to occur on flat, rounded and/or convex areas of bone (e.g. limb shafts)[14]; factors present in the burial environment that could potentially mimic metal or flint marks; associated with other environmental damage (e.g. pressure features, plastic deformation)[15]
Faunal	Tooth	Scores /furrows	**Rodent score/furrow** Short, flat, round bottomed grooves[16]. **Carnivore score/furrow** Broad rounded or 'u'-shaped cross section[17]. **Rodent and carnivore score/furrow** Follow the contour of the bone; broad; frequently occur in parallel groups; generally perpendicular orientation.	Concentrated in areas where there is the least soft tissue and the cancellous bone is less dense (e.g. epiphyseal ends of long bones)[20], associated 'scooped' or 'hollowed' out cancellous bone and splintering[21]; nutritionally meaningful locations (i.e. in regions where the bone is richest in its marrow content); located on prominent areas of bone where it is easy to latch on; often on medullar and cortical surfaces and/or thickness[22].
Faunal	Tooth	Pits	Bowl shaped interiors; 'u'-shaped cross-sections; evidence for internal crushing; rarely accompanied by microstriations but when present they are broad, disparate and deep[18]	
Faunal	Tooth	Punctures	Depressed fractures; roughly circular outline; sometimes stepped appearance; may contain fragments pushed inwards[19].	

(based on Behrensmeyer et al. 1986; Binford 1981; Cook 1986; Greenfield 2000; Haglund et al. 1988; Hurlbut 2000; Lyman 1994; Milner & Smith 1989; Morlan 1984; Oliver 1989, Olsen & Shipman 1988; Bunn 1981; Blumenschine & Selvaggio 1988; Bunn 1981; Blumenschine 1995; Blumenschine et al. 1996; Blumenschine & Selvaggio 1988; Bunn 1981; Shipman & Rose 1983; Walker & Long 1977). [1]Greenfield 2000:99-100; [2]Greenfield 2000:99-100; Walker & Long 1977:608-609; Shipman and Rose 1983: 68-69; [3]Hurlbut 2000:7; [4]Lyman 1994: 298; [5]Oliver 1989:93; [6]Behrensmeyer et al. 1986:770; [7]Potts & Shipman 1981:577; Shipman 1981; [8]Blumenschine & Slevaggio 1988:764-765; Blumenschine et al. 1996:496; Potts & Shipman 1981:577; [9]Blumenschine & Slevaggio 1988:764-765; Blumenschine 1995:29; [10]Blumenschine & Selvaggio 1988:764; [11]Blumenschine et al. 1996:496; [12]Blumenschine & Selvaggio 1991:23, 28; [13]Blumenschine & Selvaggio 1988:765; Cook 1986:282-283; Olsen & Shipman 1988:543; Shipman & Rose 1983; [14]Behrensmeyer et al. 1986: 770; Olsen & Shipman 1988: 544; [15]Cook 1986:282; Oliver 1989:93; [16]Bunn 1981:575; [17]Bunn 1981:575; [18]Binford 1981; Blumenschine 1995:29; Blumenschine et al. 1996:496; Bunn 1981; Morlan 1984; [19]Blumenschine 1995:29; Shipman 1981:366; [20]Blumenschine 1988; Haglund et al. 1988; Milner and Smith 1989; [21]Binford 1981; Haglund et al. 1988; [22]Blumenschine et al. 1996:4

The matter of intentionality

Shipman and Rose (1983:62) argued that a cut mark is only evidence that a sharp artefact was used to remove tissue; it is not evidence *per se* for the intention behind the activity. To this end, the importance of considering factors such as the location (e.g. in the region of muscle attachments) and orientation (transverse or parallel to the long axis) of cut marks, as well as associated features (e.g. peri-mortem fracture) has been stressed (Hurlbut 2000). In seeking to do this, however, it should be remembered that while activities such as defleshing and disarticulation may be intentional, the actual marks left on the bones are *unintentional* – they are the by-products of the activities and the intentions (Hambleton, pers comm.).

Conspicuous versus inconspicuous features

Some features may not be identified unless elements are examined microscopically or with a hand lens under strong, low incidence light. Blumenschine and Marean (1993) found that the majority of tooth marks on experimentally gnawed animal bones were inconspicuous, that is, not visible to the naked eye. It has subsequently been argued that the systematic dedicated examination of elements under magnification is essential if surface features are to be studied accurately (Blumenschine et al. 1996). Recent work on Bronze Age remains recovered from the palaeo-channel at Eton (O'Sullivan 2001) supports this argument and suggests that features could be missed unless surfaces are inspected microscopically (Fig. 3). This issue is part of a wider debate over the microscopic analysis of features. It has been argued that identification and interpretation can only be properly explored by the application of scanning electron microscopy because light microscopes have a poor depth of field, limited magnification, and the resolution of three-dimensional structures is inferior (Shipman 1981:360-1). Conversely, others argue that this level of analysis is not always necessary (Bunn 1981) and that SEM analysis may bias the identification and interpretation of features because it ignores the overall context of a modification (Blumenschine et al. 1996).

This is supported by controlled tests which have reported a 99% success rate in identifying known actor and effector when elements are examined with a hand lens and a light microscope (Blumenschine et al. 1996).

This aspect of surface feature analysis requires more detailed testing, with greater emphasis placed on questions such as whether specialists have the time for this level of analysis, and how much will be missed if specimens are not examined at this level.

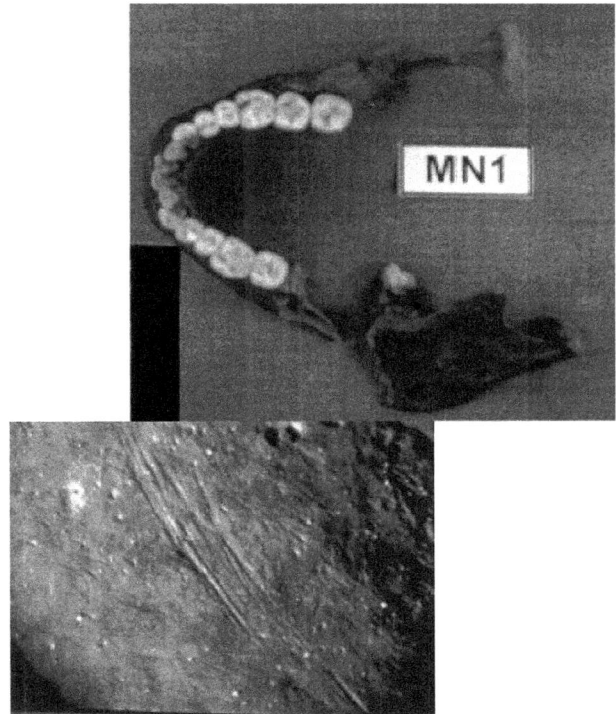

Figure 3. When the lingual surface of the right ascending ramus of this mandible (top) was examined microscopically (bottom), a patch of unidirectional superior-inferior striations were visible. Their features are suggestive of scrape marks made with a tool whilst the bone was still fresh (O'Sullivan, 2001:44); they have 'v'-shaped profiles, smooth margins and cut into the surface of the bone but, unlike cut marks, they are shallow and their margins are not sharp. They were not identified macroscopically. *(Photographed by I. O'Sullivan).*

Surface Features as Part of an Integrated Approach to Modification Studies: An Example from Fishmonger Swallet, Alveston, Gloucestershire

Excavation at Fishmonger Swallet by archaeologists in 2000, and prior to this by the Hades Caving Club, yielded an assemblage of late Iron Age/early Roman disarticulated human bones that represent a minimum number of six adults (1,940+/-40BP; Cal BP 1,980 to 1,820) (Cox, 2001). One of the elements, a fragment of right femoral shaft (Fig. 4), was longitudinally split, with fracture margins characteristic of peri-mortem breakage, including a helical break at the distal end (Villa & Mahieu 1991). The bone was blackened by bacterial activity from within the burial environment, thus modern fractures were easy to identify (Cox 2001; Fig. 4).

Longitudinally split fragments are described by Villa and Mahieu (1991:43) as 'elongate splinters' and may be indicative of a long bone shaft being split by humans for marrow extraction (Cox 2001). Longitudinal breaks are not unique to this activity but are also a natural response of diaphyseal bones to transverse sediment pressure in which the fracture front follows the orientation of the haversian systems and collagen fibre bundles (Trinkhaus, 1985:206). Longitudinal breakage has also been documented as a part of weathering (Behrensmeyer, 1978 Table 5, in Buikstra and Ubelaker 1994) and carnivore scavenging processes (Binford 1981). Helical fracture patterns are not confined to anthropogenic behaviour,as demonstrated by controlled experiments examining fracture patterns resulting from animal trampling (Haynes 1986).

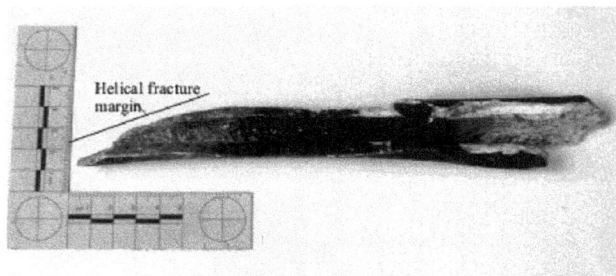

Figure 4. Longitudinal split femur fragment from Fishmonger Swallet, Alveston. *(M. Cox).*

The fracture morphology of the femur fragment is not evidence alone for deliberate breakage by humans; it is only evidence that the fracture occurred when the bone was fresh (Johnson, 1985). Deliberate breakage by humans can only be identified if the fracture is accompanied by surface features, namely percussion marks (Blumenschine 1995; Blumenschine & Selvaggio, 1988). In order to explore actor, effector and determine whether the fracture was deliberate, a detailed macroscopic and microscopic examination of the bone for surface features was undertaken by employing the methodology described above. In this particular instance, all observations were made using a 10x hand lens and a stereo light microscope.

Three primary groups of surface features were identified on the fragment, and all of these have peri-mortem characteristics (Fig. 5). The first group, located on the medio-posterior aspect and very proximal end of zone 6 (the middle portion of the diaphysis), is represented by three unidirectional, sub-parallel, elongate, grooves (ranging from about 4mm to 7mm long and about 1mm wide). These grooves have a transverse orientation in relation to the long axis of the bone and have blunt, straight margins. They cut into the bone and have 'v' shaped profiles that are shallow and wide. They lack the clean internal appearance of marks made with metal tools and they have no distinct apex. One wall is comparatively steep, the other comparatively sloped. Both walls tend to be concave and both contain uni-directional sub-parallel striations that run in the same direction as the main groove. They tend to be more apparent on one wall than the other and give an overall impression of shallow interconnected grooves (Long & White 1977:608). Sub-parallel transverse micro-striations flank the outside

margins of the two outer grooves. These features are consistent with a diagnosis of cuts made with a stone tool (Table 3).

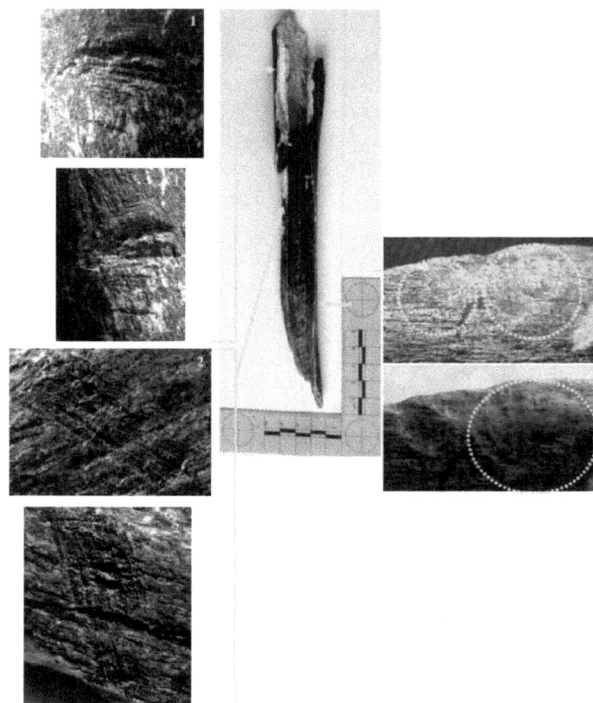

Figure 5. Surface alterations on the Fishmonger Swallet femur fragment: 1. Cut marks (two views), 2. Percussion marks (two views), 3. Scoop marks (two views). *(Photographed by L. Loe).*

Just below these, is a deeper striation which cuts into the bone, has a sharp and narrow 'v'-shaped profile and runs obliquely from superior left to inferior right. This also has straight margins of which one is comparatively sharp, the other comparatively flaked. Unlike the grooves, this feature is uniform and has a well-defined apex. Sub-parallel micro-striations are present on the surface of one wall and the uniform depth and spacing of these, may indicate that they represent a cut mark made by a metal tool (Table 3). However, this surface feature also has an abraded, or 'unclean', internal appearance, indicating that it could represent a cut mark made with a stone tool (Greenfield 2000).

The second group comprises a dense patch of superficial, uni-directional, parallel, micro-striations. These occupy an oblique orientation, running from superior right to inferior left. These are located on the middle portion of zone six on the medio-posterior surface. They are very straight and are within 5mm from the fracture margin. Their morphology and location, within 5mm of the fracture margin, are consistent with striations resulting from percussion abrasion (Blumenschine & Selvaggio 1988). It is unlikely that these represent cut marks because they are shallow and narrow. Tooth scores are unlikely because, although shallow, they are not broad, do not have a 'u' shaped profile and are not located on a prominent area of the bone where it is easy for a rodent to latch on. Sediment abrasion is unlikely because this tends to result in striations that are multi-directional and have an uneven thickness, whereas these are transverse, unidirectional and even. Scraping marks are possible because they are dense, straight, parallel, and shallow. However, such marks are usually orientated parallel to the longitudinal axis of the bone (Blumenschine & Selvaggio 1991), and is not the in the present example.

The last group of surface features is located on the middle portion of zone six on the lateral aspect of the shaft and is represented by two shallow sub-circular scooped areas which are polished and smooth. These may have occurred as a result of removing the periosteum to facilitate fracturing the bone, their location adjacent to the fracture margin strengthening this interpretation (Outram, pers comm.). This practice has been documented among the Nunamiut of north central Alaska who, by scraping bone with a stone tool, performed this task when the intended method of breakage was through the central area of the bone shaft (Binford 1978:153). The Fishmonger scoops are highly polished suggesting that, in this instance, removal was undertaken with a bladed instrument.

To summarise, the morphological features of these three groups most closely resemble those of:

1. cut marks (possibly with stone and metal implements),
2. percussion abrasion, and
3. defleshing.

Based on this evidence, it may be hypothesised that in this case the actor was human and the effector was a metal and/or stone tool. Intentionality may be implied because of the combination of cut marks and fracture patterns and the occurrence of a longitudinal break and percussion abrasion.

The level of accuracy with which this interpretation may be regarded rests on the broader context of the features (see above, page 8 and Table 3). This is the subject of further work that is examining the entire human and animal bone assemblages recovered from the swallet. Preliminary observations, however, are possible. For example, the first group of features is located in an area of attachment for *M. pectineus*, indicating that they may be associated with its removal (Cox 2001). Further, if the characteristic features of percussion striations are given consideration (Table 3), then the second group of features would seem to fulfil these by their association with a peri-mortem fracture margin, and their presence on a large mid-shaft fragment. Further, no surface features that

may be attributed to faunal and/or environmental activity were identified. Therefore, minimal or no exposure prior to deposition and/or exposure to an unstable burial environment is implied.

Conclusions

Peri and post-mortem surface alteration analysis, when applied to the analysis of fracture morphologies and fragmentation patterns, maximises the potential to accurately interpret modified assemblages. Until further experimental research is undertaken (especially that which takes the British burial context more fully into account), a conservative approach to this type of analysis is imperative. To this end, the morphological and metrical features of all surface alterations should be objectively scored and assigned to a most likely actor and effector. This information should be approached from an holistic perspective. Thus, in addition to studying fracture morphologies and fragmentation patterns, factors such as how an assemblage was excavated, conditions of the excavation, the processing of the material, its history as part of a museum collection and any associated faunal material must all be considered.

Acknowledgements

The authors would like to thank Irene O'Sullivan for allowing us to use her illustration shown in Figure 3. Dr Mary Lewis and Dr Ellen Hambleton are thanked for their comments on previous versions of this paper. This research is funded by HEFCE's Human Resources Initiative.

Literature Cited

Anderson, T (1996) Cranial weapon injuries from Saxon Dover. *International Journal of Osteoarchaeology* 6: 10-14.

Behrensmeyer AK (1978) Taphonomic and ecologic information from bone weathering. *Palaeobiology* 4:150-162.

Behrensmeyer AK, Gordon KD, and Yanagi GT (1986) Trampling as a cause of bone surface damage and pseudo-cut marks. *Nature* 319: 768-771.

Binford LR (1978) *Nunamiut Ethnoarchaeology.* New York: Academic Press.

Binford L (1981) *Bones: Ancient Men and Modern Myths.* New York: Academic Press.

Blumenschine RJ (1988) An experimental model of the timing of hominid and carnivore influence on archaeological bone assemblages. *Journal of Archaeological Science* 15: 483-502.

Blumenschine RJ (1995) Percussion marks, tooth marks, and experimental determinations of the timing of hominid and carnivore access to long bones at FLK Zinjanthropus, Olduvai Gorge, Tanzania. *Journal of Human Evolution* 29: 21-51.

Blumenshine RJ and Marean CW (1993) A carnivore's view of archaeological bone assemblages. In J Hudson (ed.): *From Bones to Behaviour. Ethnoarchaeological and Experimental Interpretation of Faunal Remains.* Center for Archaeological Investigations: South Illinois University at Carbondale, USA. Occasional Paper No. 21: 273-300.

Blumenschine RJ, Marean CW and Capaldo SD (1996) Blind tests of inter-analyst correspondence and accuracy in the identification of cut marks, percussion marks, and carnivore tooth marks on bone surfaces. *Journal of Archaeological Science* 23: 493-507.

Blumenschine RJ and Selvaggio MM (1988) Percussion marks on bone surfaces as a new diagnostic of hominid behaviour. *Nature* 333: 763-765.

Blumenschine RJ and Selvaggio MM (1991) On the marks of marrow bone processing by hammerstones and hyenas: their anatomical patterning and archaeological implications. In JD Clark (ed.): *Cultural Beginnings. Approaches to Understanding early Hominid Life-ways in the African Savanna.* Dr Rudolf Habelt GMBH: Bonn. Band 19: 17-32.

Boylston A, Knusel, CJ, and Roberts CA (2000) Investigation of a Romano-British rural ritual in Bedford, England. *Journal of Archaeological Science* 27:241-254.

Brain CK (1981) *The Hunters or the Hunted? An Introduction to African Cave Taphonomy.* Chicago: University of Chicago Press.

Brothwell D (1976) Further evidence of bone chewing by ungulates: The sheep of North Ronaldsay, Orkney. *Journal of Anthropological Science* 3:179-182.

Buikstra JE and Ubelaker D (eds.) (1994) *Standards for Data Collection from Human Skeletal Remains.* Fayetteville, AK: Arkansas Archaeological Survey, Research Seminar Series No. 44.

Bunn HT (1981) Archaeological evidence for meat eating by plio-pleistocene hominids from Koobi Fora and Olduvai Gorge. *Nature* 291: 574-577.

Cook J (1986) Marked human bones from Gough's cave, Somerset. *Proceedings of the Bristol Spelaeology Society* 17: 275-285.

Cox M (2001) T*he Human Skeletal Remains Assessment Report.* Time Team Series VIII. Fishmonger Swallet, Alveston, Gloucestershire. Unpublished report.

Greenfield HJ (2000) The origins of metallurgy in the central Balkans based on the Analysis of cut marks on animal bones. *Environmental Archaeology* 5: 93-106.

Haglund WB, Reay DT and Swindler, DR (1988) Tooth mark artefacts and survival of bones in animal scavenged human remains. *Journal of Forensic Sciences* 33: 985-997.

Harman M, Molleson T and Price JL (1981) Burials, bodies and beheadings in Romano-British and Anglo-Saxon cemeteries. *Bulletin of the British Museum Natural History (Geology)* 35: 145-188.

Haynes GR (1986) Spiral fractures and cut mark-mimics in non-cultural elephant bone assemblages. *Current Research in the Pleistocene* 3: 45-46.

Hurlburt SA (2000) The taphonomy of cannibalism: a review of anthropogenic bone modification in the American Southwest. *International Journal of Osteoarchaeology* 10: 4-26.

Johnson E (1985) Current developments in bone technology. In *Advances in archaeological Method and Theory.* Schiffer MB. (ed.) London: Academic Press Inc; 8:157-235.

Knüsel CJ and Outram AK (2004) Fragmentation: The zonation method applied to fragmented human remains from archaeological and forensic contexts. Environmental Archaeology. *The Journal of Human Palaeoecology* 9: 85-97

Lovejoy CO and Heiple KG (1981) Analysis of fractures in skeletal populations with an example from the Libben site, Ottawa Country, Ohio. *American Journal of Physical Anthropology* 55: 529-541.

Lyman RL (1994) *Vertebrate Taphonomy.* Cambridge Manuals in Archaeology. Cambridge University Press. Cambridge.

Mays S and Steele J. (1996) A mutilated human skull from Roman St Albans, Hertfordshire, England. *Antiquity* 70: 155-61.

Mckinley J (1992) A skull wound and possible trepanation from a Roman cemetery at Baldock, Hertfordshire. *International Journal of Osteoarchaeology* 2: 337-40.

Milner GR and Smith VG (1989) Carnivore alteration of human bone from a late prehistoric site. *American Journal of Physical Anthropology* 79:43-49.

Molleson T and Cox M (1988) A Neonate with cut bones from Poundbury Camp, 4th century AD, England. *Bulletin de la Societie Royale Belge D'Anthropologie et de Prehistoire* 99:53-9.

Morlan RE (1984) Toward the definition of criteria for the recognition of artificial bone alterations. *Quaternary Research* 22:160-171.

Murphy E (2003) *Cut marks on a prehistoric mandible from Millin Bay, Co. Down.* Palaeopathology Association Irish Section News No. 6.

Novak SA (2000) Battle-related trauma. In V Fiorato, A Boylston, and C Knüsel (eds.): *Blood Red Roses. The Archaeology of a Mass Grave from the Battle of Towton AD 1461.* Oxford: Oxbow Books; 77-102.

Oliver JS (1989) Analogues and site context: bone damages from Shield Trap cave (24CB91), Carbon County, Montana, U.S.A. In R Bonnichsen and MH Sorg (eds.): *Bone Modification.* Maine: Center for the Study of the First Americans.

Olsen SL and Shipman P (1988) Surface modification on bone: trampling versus butchery. *Journal of Archaeological Science* 15: 535-553.

O'Sullivan MI (2001) *An analysis of possible anthropogenic alteration of human bones recovered from Eton Rowing Lake, South Buckinghamshire, U.K.* Unpublished MSc dissertation, University of Bournemouth.

Parry LA (1952) The Ovingdean skull with some notes on prehistoric trephining. *Sussex Archaeological Collections* 90: 40-50.

Potts R and Shipman P (1981) Cutmarks made by stone tools on bones from Olduvai Gorge, Tanzania. *Nature* 291: 577-580.

Roberts CA and McKinley J (2003) A review of British trepanations in antiquity focusing on funerary context to explain their occurrence. In S Finger, R Arnott, and CUM Smith (eds.): *Trepanation. History, Discovery, Method.* Lisse, Swets and Zeitlinger Publishers; 55-78.

Schulting RJ and Wysocki M (2002) Cranial trauma in the British earlier Neolithic *Past* 41:4-6.

Shipman P (1981) Applications of scanning electron microscopy to taphonomic problems. In AE Cantwell, JB Griffin, and NA Rothschild (eds.): *The Research Potential of Anthropological Museum Collections.* New York: Annals of the New York Academy of Science; 376: 357-385.

Shipman P and Rose J (1983) Early hominid hunting, butchering, and carcass – processing behaviours: approaches to the fossil record. *Journal of Anthropological Archaeology* 2: 57-98.

Smith MJ and Brickley MB (2004) Analysis and interpretation of flint toolmarks found on bones from West Tump long barrow, Gloucestershire. *International Journal of Osteoarchaeology* 14: 18-33.

Sutcliff AJ (1973) Similarity of bones and antlers gnawed by deer to human artefacts. *Nature* 246: 428-430.

Trinkaus E (1985) Cannibalism and burial at Krapina. *Journal of Human Evolution* 14:203-216.

Villa P and Mahieu E (1991) Breakage patterns of human long bones. *Journal of Human Evolution* 21: 27-48.

Wakely J (1997) Identification and analysis of violent and non-violent head injuries in osteoarchaeological material. In J Carman (ed.): *Material Harm. Archaeological Studies of War and Violence.* Glasgow: Cruithne Press; 24-46.

Walker PL and Long JC (1977) An experimental study of the morphological characteristics of tool marks. *American Antiquity* 42: 605-616.

Wells C (1974) Probable trepanation of five early Saxon skulls. *Antiquity* 48: 298-302.

Wells C (1981) The human burials. In A McWhirr, L Viner, C Wells (eds.): *Romano-British Cemeteries at Cirencester. Vol. 2. Cirencester Excavations.* Cirencester: Corinium Museum; 135-202.

Wysocki M and Whittle A (2000) Diversity, lifestyles and rites: new biological and archaeological evidence from British earlier Neolithic mortuary assemblages. *Antiquity* 74: 591-601.

New perspectives on preservation of the dead: a review of the underlying physico-chemical principles involved
or
Preservation of the dead — a thwarted bacterium's view

William J White, C Chem, FRSC

Centre for Human Bioarchaeology
The Museum of London
150 London Wall, London EC2Y 5HN
bwhite@museumoflondon.org.uk
Tel: +44(0) 207 814 5649; Fax: +44(0) 0870 444 3853

Abstract

The list of excellent publications on the archaeology and palaeopathology of mummified human bodies continues to grow. Unfortunately, rarely can space be found to do more than touch upon the scientific principles responsible for the preservation of soft tissue. In general, it is acknowledged that it is primarily the host's commensal bacteria that give rise to putrefaction. Nonetheless, the ways of inhibition of bacterial growth and enzymatic activity that occur during mummification, whether spontaneous, artificial or concerted, are often over-simplified. It is frequently a multifactorial process. Thus, one may see it stated that there are three, four or five preservative principles, presumably acting both independently and mutually exclusively. This may be valid if the preservation of foodstuffs is regarded as a suitable model for the mechanism of bacteriostasis. From the viewpoint of microbial inhibition, however, the number of available biocidal factors runs into double figures. Accordingly, there is a need for the general principles of soft tissue preservation to be re-defined. In this systematic review the bacteriology and enzymology involved in the preservation of the human dead, are explored, with some case studies and evaluation of the predictive potential.

Keywords

Adipocere, Bacteria, Commensals, Enzyme, Inhibition, Multi-factorial Preservation, Taphonomy

Introduction

Successful mummification is dependent upon the inhibition of the multiplication of micro-organisms. No systematic review encompassing all the theoretically possible inhibitory factors has yet appeared, though, even though forty years have passed since the pioneering approach first made to the problem (Evans 1963). Thus, it is possible to see it declared that up to five preservative factors are available (eg. Aufderheide 2003, 42-3). Honourable mention ought to be given to the recent elegant system of classification into four "conditions conducive to soft issue preservation" (Chamberlain & Parker Pearson 200: 14-5). These classes: 'cold', 'dry', 'wet' and 'sterile' are not intended to be exclusive; instead each is a portmanteau term within which multiple preservative mechanisms may be in operation. Most reviews tend to oversimplify the picture as the total number of preservative principles available greatly exceeds the above by at least a factor of two. The chemistry and bacteriology involved in preservation will be reviewed here, with an emphasis on the fact that the mummification involved is often multifactorial in origin. Case studies will be presented to exemplify this.

Chemistry of Putrefaction

There is nothing inherent in highly-organised tissue causing it to decompose spontaneously, merely because it is no longer animated. When homeostasis ceases, upon the death of an organism, there is no spontaneous tendency to a cascade of chemical reactions for the decomposition of complex compounds into simpler ones. Instead it occurs in stages, a controlled step-wise degradation of complex molecules, ultimately into simple organic and inorganic compounds. The intermediate products from all stages in this retrosynthetic process are each thermodynamically stable and chemically inert. Each individual chemical transition requires overcoming an energy barrier. As suitable energy sources usually are unavailable the requisite chemical alterations are not favoured. What, then, is the driving force for the chemical changes invoked in putrefaction? In certain chemical reactions the energy barrier can be over-ridden *via* catalysis, using enzymes. Thus, each step in the reaction sequence is mediated by specific extra-cellular enzymes secreted primarily by the commensal bacteria.[1] Enzymes of non-bacterial origin have been implicated in early post-mortem decomposition *via* 'auto-digestion' of certain organs although the process (autolysis) appears haphazard (Garland 1989).[2]

The thermodynamic stability of the body tissues can be demonstrated by consideration of the fate of "germ-free" rats and mice. When individuals of these germ-free strains die (or, more appositely, are killed during medical research) their corpses do not putrefy (Davis et al. 1972). A similar situation pertains with regard to stillborn children, who remain sterile in the microbial sense (Chamberlain & Parker Pearson 2001: 14).

The onset of decay in intact cadavers depends upon efficient operation of the catalysts secreted by the putrefactive bacteria. Factors capable of inhibiting microbial activity are summarised in Table 1. An evaluation of their operations follows, with examples in which the predicted inhibition has been realised in mummification, whether spontaneous or deliberate.

Table 1: Factors influencing the growth and multiplication of bacteria: their applicability to soft tissue preservation, whether spontaneous or deliberate (Duguid et al., 1978; Parry and Pawsey 1990)

FACTOR	SPONTANEOUS	ARTIFICIAL
Atmosphere	X	X
Dehydration	X	X
Temperature	X	X
pH	X	X
Osmosis	X	X
Antibiotics	?	X
Protoplasmic	X	X
Irradiation	--	X
Mechanical	--	--
Pressure	--	--
Nutrition	X	X

Key:- X = occurrence -- = unknown

[1] The situation described concerns the early stages in the instigation of decomposition, the identity of the enzyme concerned being specific to the substrate and micro-organism involved. Evisceration represents an intervention strategy that lowers the risk of decay by removing the bulk of the commensal bacteria along with their habitat. Later the enzymes supplied by opportunistic bacteria from the exterior environment or from the larvae of any scavenging arthropods can also come into play. Moreover, the exclusion of oxygen is important in its own right, as non-enzymatic oxidative secondary reactions are equally inimical to soft tissue preservation.

[2] A major consideration is that autolysis of specialised organs may occur under the influence of the enzymes secreted therein, the lysosymes (Aufderheide 2003, 318- 321). Despite this, there are numerous instances of specialised structures such as eyes and brains robustly having avoided severe biodeterioration and liquefaction (Chamberlain and Parker Pearson 2001, 49, 88). The author was present during recent excavations in a London cemetery, in use from 1792 to c. 1850. Of over 700 skeletons recovered from water-logged wooden coffins at least 30 still had the brain present, soft but not noticeably shrunken. Unfortunately circumstances precluded histological or other investigation.

Factors Influencing the Growth and Multiplication of Bacteria

1 Modified Atmosphere

Aerobic bacteria require oxygen, of course, and anaerobic bacteria carbon dioxide but other microbes are less discriminating ('facultative'). Taphonomy is of great importance as burial conditions may control the nature of gases in the local environment. Hermetically-sealed coffins, water-logged deposits lacking dissolved gases, deliberate sealing of the body in its coffin with pitch or resins or sealing the shroud with a layer of beeswax and so on provide microclimates in which the gases necessary for microbial respiration are absent or readily depleted.

2 Desiccation

Water constitutes an extremely high proportion of bacterial cell wall, up to 80% (Parry & Pawsley 1990: 31). It follows that if water is removed from the substrate the growth of bacteria will be halted. Here the physical dimensions of the cadaver are important, exsiccation being a more efficient process when the ratio of the surface area of the body to its volume is high, as in a juvenile of the species. The same applies to the cognate process of preservation by *freeze-drying*, the removal of water by sublimation from the frozen state (Chamberlain & Parker Pearson 200: 196). In spontaneous preservation of the dead, desiccation is known both in arid zones and in temperate areas under suitable undisturbed well ventilated situations. The distribution of exsiccated mummies is wide, from the western and south-western areas of the USA, Mexico, littoral Peru and Chile, Spain, Southern France, Italy, Austria, the British Isles, the Middle East and China (Vreeland 1998: 155-7; Aufderheide 2003: 80-4, 88-91, 164-170, 183, 193-202, 260-271; Pike 2004). Desiccation has been used widely in deliberate mummification, whether artificial or assisted.

3 Control of Temperature

The viability and growth of bacteria are subject to control, depending upon the ambient temperature. Bacteria thrive within an optimum temperature range of 5 to 45 degrees Celsius (Parry & Pawsley 1990, 35). Certain bacteria have evolved to survive extremes of temperature (thermophiles) but these generally are not the ones implicated in decomposition of soft tissue. Fire-drying as part of the funerary process is strictly a means of accelerated *desiccation*. In "smoking" human bodies it is not the high temperatures reached that influence preservation so much as the chemical changes induced by exposure to the colloidal distillate in the fumes (see below).

At the lower end of the temperature range a different situation obtains. Cooling retards the growth of bacteria.

Preservation by freezing is also subject to acceleration by a high surface-area-to-volume ratio, as discussed above. Thus, preservation of juveniles tends to be enhanced with respect to adults of the species. This holds also with the Quaternary fauna preserved in the permafrost of Alaska and Siberia, wherein the young of the megafauna such as *Mammuthus primigenius* are better preserved than the adults and the small mammals in superior condition to the extinct megafauna (Zimmerman and Tedford 1976; White 1982; Guthrie 1990: 16-20).

4 Hydrogen ion concentration

The commensal microflora grow best under neutral or slightly alkaline conditions, with an optimum pH range 7.2 to 7.6 (Parry & Pawsley 1990: 35-6). Highly alkaline conditions are lethal to bacteria but no burial deposits with a high pH are known. The mineral natron, native sodium carbonate as used in ancient Egyptian mummification, is formally an alkali but its efficiency in embalming is dependent chiefly upon its other chemical properties (Peck 1998: 28-32). Similarly, the preservative effect of quicklime (calcium oxide) is based not merely upon its mild alkalinity but primarily upon its desiccant properties (Mendelsohn 1940: 141).

The peat bogs of northern Europe, known for the remarkable preservation of human bodies and faunal remains, are acidic, pH 3.2 to 6.5 (Painter 1995: 90). However, it is now known that bog bodies owe their remarkable state of preservation to taphonomy in which a number of preservative factors are acting in concert, not merely low pH and anoxic waterlogged conditions. Several types of artificial means of preservation of the dead, however, do make use of the low pH effect, just as in the analogous "pickling" of foods (Coultate 1984: 179-82). Thus, in medieval Europe the bodies of royalty, the nobility, the higher clergy and state criminals often were preserved by marination in a "pickle", the major ingredient of which was vinegar (White 1985). Exhumations have revealed preserved medieval corpses lying in such an infusion. These include a fourteenth century knight at Danbury, Essex, and Humphrey, Duke of Gloucester (d1447) in St Albans Abbey (White 1985: 375; White 1998; Chamberlain & Parker Pearson 2001: 26-27).

5 Osmosis

Bacteria possess a cell wall that constitutes a semi-permeable cytoplasmic membrane. They are therefore extremely sensitive to osmotic effects and the local application of hydrophilic agents will draw water from the interior of the bacterial cells, causing their death by plasmolysis. Here the mechanism of osmosis is profoundly different from simple desiccation. A wide range of hygroscopic agents can promote preservation by osmosis but few are known to cause spontaneous preservation. Common salt (sodium chloride) is highly

effective in this regard, and is exploited in the preservation of food, especially meat, for long-term storage. However, apart from anecdotal accounts of the preservation of dead salt miners, or certain burials in saline soils (Aufderheide 2003: 171) perhaps the best spontaneous example known is the perfectly preserved cadaver of a woolly rhinoceros (*Coelodonta antiquitatis*) in a salt-saturated deposit in Poland (Novack et al. 1930).

The osmotic effect was chiefly made use of in artificial preservation in ancient and medieval times, using salts, sugars, honey or alcohol for processing the dead (White 1985: 374). Of these, alcohol possesses additional germicidal activity, whereas honey from certain sources appears also to have antimicrobial properties owing to a high peroxide content (Willix et al. 1992; Subrahmanyam 1993). Although tradition has it that the corpse of Alexander the Great was preserved in honey, doubts have been expressed as to whether this commodity is capable of preserving an intact adult human body (Aufderheide 2003: 46-8). However, there are accounts of the preservation of the bodies of juveniles in jars of honey in Egypt (Hamilton-Paterson & Andrews 1978: 61).

6 Antibiotics

Antibiotics act by interfering with bacterial cell wall synthesis. Despite more than half a century of antibiotic drug use the prediction that this would lead to an increased prevalence of soft tissue preservation among those who died while on a course of treatment has not been borne out by experience (Chamberlain & Parker Pearson 2001: 19). However, some aromatic spices have been shown to possess a natural antibiotic. These include cinnamon, cassia, cloves, cumin, mustard, nutmeg, peppercorn, ginger, myrrh and aloes, which were used in embalming in antiquity (Billing & Sherman 1998).[3]

7 Protoplasmic poisons

The ions of certain metals and pseudometallic elements are toxic toward bacteria. These include copper, silver, zinc, mercury, arsenic, antimony and lead. Spontaneous preservation by this means is known to occur, most

---

[3] One of the purposes of embalming the deceased was that the body could be maintained in a recognisable condition were it necessary for the fact of the death to be broadcast publicly, as in the expiry of a medieval monarch (White 1985, 373). A somewhat different treatment obtained if the interment of the deceased was to be delayed for a longer period. Thus, the bodies of those who died far from home required preservative treatment if it was intended that they be repatriated for burial.

Here management was *via* the so-called '*mos teutonicus*'. The corpse was dismembered and then boiled in portions to separate the soft tissue from the bones. The bones could be reunited with the boiled flesh in a single container (or be buried separately) but the soft tissue would be preserved by steeping in spices and any material intended for repatriation then was ready to be transported (White 1985, 375, Litten 1991, 37, Maffart et al., 2004, 71). Similarly, the decapitated heads of executed traitors would be boiled with salt and spices then treated with pitch, when intended for display in prominent public places.

spectacularly perhaps in the body of a thousand-year old copper miner in Chile (Vreeland 1998: 182). Bodies are often found well preserved in zinc or zinc-lined coffins, particularly the skin which is leather-like and "corified" or "corylised" (Torre and Cardellini 1981; Torre, et al. 1982). Preserved bodies have been encountered in the presence of mercury or its salts but it is not always evident whether the observed preservation was intentional (Mendelson 1940: 11; Yamada 1990; Peng 1995; Fornaciari & Capasso 1996: 198). Saturation of the tissues is not required for, even if present in only very small traces, the metal ions can promote the preservation of soft tissue by de-activation of the putrefactive enzymes involved, cf. catalyst "poisoning" (Aufderheide 2003: 306). The deliberate use of inorganic poisons is rare in embalmic practice, although arsenic was so used in North America in the nineteenth century (Mendelsohn 1940: 13-14; Aufderheide 2003: 304-5). Several examples exist from the late 19th century of bodies preserved by means of arterial injection of a solution of arsenious acid (Aufderheide 2003: 85-88). Protoplasmic poisons also include phenolic compounds and aldehydes in the complex chemical gallimaufry to which bodies (or foods) are exposed during the "smoking" process (Coultate 1984: 183-4).

8 Irradiation

Surfaces can be sterilised using ultra-violet radiation (uv), but the incident radiation received from the Sun lacks sufficient intensity to promote the preservation of an exposed corpse and macroscopic scavengers usually cause mechanical damage at an early stage.[4] There is no known example of spontaneous preservation of the dead by means of uv, microwave irradiation nor nuclear radiation. Nevertheless, gamma radiation has found some practical application in this field, having been used to cure a fungal infection in the mummy of *Ramesses II,* using a cobalt-60 source and resulting in a renewed state of sterility (Aufderheide 2003: 312).

9 Vibration

Metabolism and growth of bacteria are subject to arrest by severe mechanical disturbance. The stresses caused by vibration and ultrasound disrupt contents of the bacterial cell. It is difficult to cite circumstances under which preservation by these means might occur spontaneously and even if it did then the mechanical vibration or sonication would require constant renewal or some form of antisepsis to maintain the sterile state. Accordingly

there is no known practical application in embalming practice.[5]

10 Pressure

At one extreme, that of zero pressure, one is dealing with a vacuum and this involves a different preservative factor (anaeorobiosis above). As to the effect of elevated pressure no examples are known (Parry & Pawsley 1990: 39).

11 Nutrition

Ostensibly the cadaver presents a ready-meal to micro-organisms. The intact body itself may seem to present a good source of nourishment but conditions may prevent its utilisation. Bacteria require nutrients in liquid form. If the protein of the soft tissue is denatured or coagulated by any means, it is rendered insoluble and bacterial nutrition thereby is hindered. The principal mechanism for the preservation of bog bodies depends on such a mechanism.. Natural tannic and humic acids and the complex saccharides (sugars) in the sphagnum moss react with protein *via* a variant of the 'Maillard Reaction' to produce a thickened mass that is insoluble and therefore unavailable as a nutrient medium for bacteria (Painter 1995: 95).

The tissue preservative action of alcohols depends chiefly upon the precipitation of a complex of tissue protein with an alcohol. Tissues 'fixed' in this manner are rendered far less soluble and therefore resistant to microbially-mediated degradation. In modern embalming practice aldehydes have several roles but one of the most important lies in condensation reactions that increase the cross-linking of proteins *via* their free amino groups, hence lowering solubility.

12 Adipocere Formation

This is a special case involving nutrition or lack of it. Microbial saponification of the body fat results in a complex mixture of fatty acids and their hydroxylated analogues (Frankel 1984; Gotouda et al. 1988; Yan et al. 2001). The chemical products possess very low solubility and hence are highly resistant to further bacterial attack.

Case Studies

Oetzi: freezing, desiccation and adipocere formation?

Thirteen years after the discovery of the mummified body of the so-called 'Iceman' of the Tyrolean Alps (Oetzi) the

---

[4] When bodies lying on the surface undergo mummification this tends to occur both where scavengers are absent and the ambient bacterial count low, such as in hyperarid conditions (Chamberlain and Parker Pearson 2001, 113) or the seals and penguins preserved by freeze-drying in the Antarctic (Pewe et al., 1959, Claridge 1961).

[5] A commercial organisation in Sweden offers effectively a cold alternative to cremation. The body is frozen in liquid nitrogen, vibrated until it has disintegrated and the resultant powder freeze-dried losing about 75% of its mass (www.promessa.se/illustration_en.asp accessed January 2004).

reason(s) for the remarkable state of preservation of the body remains unresolved. Preservation by freezing alone has never been seriously proposed and some form of desiccation is generally assumed (Aufderheide 2003: 45, 314). Studies on the ultrastructure of the skin by spectroscopic methods have tended to support this mechanism yet, following GC-MS lipid analysis of tissue samples at a different laboratory, preservation solely *via* adipocere formation has been proposed (Bereuter 1999). Subsequently, these doubts cast on the contribution of dehydration to Oetzi's preservation in turn were countered by the laboratory that used Raman spectroscopy to examine tissue samples (Williams et al. 1999a, 1999b). Similar doubts as to the predominance of the desiccation mechanism had been expressed much earlier, because the body of this 1.57m-tall man still weighed c.30kg and the body was pliable rather than brittle (Spindler 1994: 54, 163). Nevertheless, the emaciated appearance of the body tended to militate against the notion of extensive aponification of adipose tissue. It has been suggested, therefore, that both preservative mechanisms could have been operating *simultaneously* (White 1999). This has been observed in other preserved bodies retrieved from glaciers Spindler 1994: 154-5). The conflicting results might be reconcilable if the two laboratories concerned were to exchange samples and attempt to reproduce one another's results (White 1999). This modest suggestion has yet to be acted upon.

Freezing, freeze-drying and embalming

Although deliberate preservation by freezing alone can be very successful and is in widespread use there appears to have been little deliberate recourse to this treatment in antiquity. In the High Andes in Peru, Chile and Argentina an assisted technique involved climatic freeze-drying (Vreeland 1998: 182). However, the famous Scythian nomad burials in the Altai owed their excellent preservation of soft tissue not to freezing alone. The observed evisceration and packing of the skin with a preservative agent, probably sodium chloride, would have arrested decay before the protective effect could come into play (Rudenko 1970; White 1980).

The Inuit bodies at Qilakitsoq, Greenland, appear to have been preserved intact by freeze-drying (Chamberlain & Parker Pearson 2001: 125-6). Genuine spontaneous preservation by freezing alone, however, is known only in interments that have been made directly into the Antarctic or Arctic permafrost (Beattie and Geiger 1987). *Egyptian mummification: desiccation, spices, oils and resins, anaerobiosis*

Evisceration or exenteration of the body (thus removing the majority of the intrinsic microflora) was of fundamental importance in ancient Egypt. Nevertheless, it has been known for nearly a century that the principal agent in ancient Egyptian mummification was natron (a naturally occurring form of sodium carbonate, containing variable amounts of sodium bicarbonate, sodium chloride and other salts), and which was applied in solid form to the naked corpse (Brier 1995; Peck 1998: 30).

Considerable programmes of animal experimentation have been performed since the time of Arthur Lucas (Peck 1998: 30-1) but the ultimate experiment was the successful embalming of a consenting human adult (Brier & Wade 1997).

Sodium carbonate was essential as it has a strong affinity for water and can exist as a stable decahydrate, following the acquisition of ten molecules of water for every molecule of the salt. Accordingly natron was used to remove water through the body's skin by osmosis. Since sodium carbonate is also strongly alkaline, during the exposure of the body to a large excess of solid natron the skin was penetrated and the epidermis was shed (Peck 1998: 32). This brought the drying agent in closer contact with the dermal layer, which then acted as a semi-permeable membrane through which water would pass outward *via* osmosis. It is thought that some Egyptian mummies were less well preserved than their contemporaries because costs had been cut by attempting to re-use natron from a previous mummification process (David 1984: 6). This miscalculation could have been circumvented by spreading the spent natron in the sun to dry. Sodium carbonate decahydrate is efflorescent in a hot, dry climate such as that of Egypt. The water in the spent natron would readily be lost, effectively reversing the equilibrium process on which the dehydration of the body depended, with anhydrous sodium carbonate being re-generated for re-use in further mummification, albeit having acquired some staining (Brier 1995: 8).

Several of the other refinements of the embalming technique were useful in reducing bacterial contamination of the mummy, such as washing the abdominal cavity with palm wine following the exenteration, then packing it with bags of natron and aromatic spices. However, only fairly recently has the treatment of the exterior of the mummified body been accorded the importance it deserves. The externally applied oils, waxes and resins presented a physico-chemical barrier, preventing re-hydration and the inoculation of the mummy with ambient micro-organisms, thus maintaining bacteriostasis and lowering the exposure to oxygen (Buckley & Evershed 2001). Similar techniques to this were used in medieval European embalming. The embalmed body was wrapped in a cerecloth (a linen shroud treated with beeswax). In the instance of the English monarch, Edward I (d1307), there is documentary evidence that the wax layer was renewed regularly up to1485 (White 1985: 373-4).

Conclusions

Post-mortem preservation is a chemical degradation process. It is not spontaneous, but is driven by catalysis.

The catalysts concerned are primarily the extra-cellular enzymes produced by the commensal bacteria . In this systematic review of preservative conditions those potentially accessible have been evaluated from first principles, as informed by enzymology and recent research. Amid the multifarious factors considered a few have yet to be found operatingly spontaneously and/or with deliberate applications. The mechanistic approach adopted has taken little account concerning whether a particular state of preservation observed was spontaneous, assisted natural, or artificial in character. Some distinction has been made where the preservation was deliberate but in the main has not been concerned with intention.

What has emerged from this prospective survey is that it is the enzymatic digestive process that requires inhibition, with chemical and physical barriers closing the nutritional pathways. Several important factors have been shown to converge upon the principle of the denial of nutrients to micro-organisms. However, the subsequent protection of the soft tissue from bacterial predation may require barrier methods to prevent re-inocculation by opportunistic microbes. and the onset of biodeterioration. There has been a primary concentration upon the influence of the commensal bacteria and the requisite enzymes released by them into the body after death has occurred. It is recognised that adventitious bacteria and enzymes from other sources may promote the biodeterioration.
Overall, it needs to be emphasised that rarely does a single mechanism prevail; the observed preservation is usually multifactorial in origin. Conversely, there may be occasions when the exact mechanisms responsible are not immediately apparent. It has long since ceased to be necessary to invoke 'miraculous preservation' (Evans 1963: 40-2); instead, spare a thought for those 'germ-free' rodents.

Literature Cited

Aufderheide AC (2003) The Scientific Study of Mummies. Cambridge: Cambridge University Press.

Beattie O and Geiger J (1987) Frozen in Time: the fate of the Franklin expedition. London: Bloomsbury.

Bereuter TL (1999) Dead, drowned and dehydrated. Chemistry in Britain 35 (8) August: 25-8.

Billing J and Sherman P (1998) Antimicrobial functions of spices. Quarterly Reviews of Biology 73: 3-49.

Brier B (1995) The use of natron in Egyptian mummification: preliminary report. Palaeopathology News 89 (June): 7-9.

Brier B and Wade RS (1997) The use of natron in Egyptian mummification: a modern experiment. Zeitschrift für Aegyptische Sprache und Altertumskunde 124: 89-100.

Buckley SA and Evershed RP (2001) Organic chemistry of embalming agents in pharoanic and Graeco-Roman mummies. Nature 413: 837-841.

Chamberlain AT and Parker Pearson M (2001) Earthly Remains: the History and Science of Preserved Human Bodies. London: British Museum Press.

Claridge GC (1961) Seal tracks in the Taylor dry valley. Nature 190: 559.

Coultate TP (1984) Food: the Chemistry of its Components. London: RSC.

David AR (1984) Mummification in Ancient Egypt. In AR David and E Tapp (ed.): Evidence Embalmed: Modern Medicine and the Mummies of Egypt. Manchester: Manchester University Press; 1-42.

Davis GL, Leffert RI, and Rantanen NW (1972) Putrefactive ethanol sources in post-mortem tissues of conventional and germ-free mice. Archives of Pathology 94: 71-4.

Duguid JP, Marmion BP, and Swain RHA (1978) Mackie & McCartney's Medical Microbiology Vol 1. 13th ed. Edinburgh and London: E&S Livingstone.

Evans WED (1963) The Chemistry of Death. Springfield: Charles C Thomas.

Fornaciari G and Capasso L (1996) Natural and artificial 13th-19th century mummies in Italy. In K Spindler, H Wilfing, E Rastbichler-Zissernig, D zur Nedden, and H Nothdurfter (ed): The Man in the Ice, Volume 3: Human Mummies, a global survey of their status and the techniques of conservation. New York: Springer-Verlag; 195-203.

Frankel EN (1984) Recent advances in the chemistry of the rancidity of fats. In AJ Bailey (ed): Recent Advances in the Chemistry of Meat. London: RSC.

Garland AN (1989) The taphonomy of inhumation burials. In CA Roberts, F Lee, and J Bintliff (ed): Burial Archaeology: current research, methods and developments. British Archaeological Reports British Series 211. Oxford: BAR Publishing; 15-37.

Gotouda H, Takatori T, Terazawa K, Nagao M, and Tarao H (1988) The mechanism of experimental adipocere formation: hydration and dehydrogenation in microbial synthesis of hydroxyl and oxo-fatty acids. Forensic Science International 37 (4): 249-57.

Guthrie RD. (1990) *Frozen Fauna of the Mammoth Steppe.* Chicago: University of Chicago Press.

Hamilton-Paterson J and Andrews C (1978) *Mummification: Life and Death in Ancient Egypt.* London: British Museum Publications.

Lane B (1992) *The Encyclopaedia of Forensic Science.* London: Hodder.

Litten J (1991) *The English Way of Death: the common funeral since 1450.* London: Robert Hale.

Mafart B, Pelletier JP, and Fixot M (2004) Post-mortem ablation of the heart: a medieval funerary practice. A case observed at the cemetery of Ganagobie Priory in the French Department of Alpes de Haut Provence. *International Journmal of Osteoarchaeology* 14: 67-73.

Mendelsohn S (1940) *Embalming Fluids: their historical Development.* New York: The Chemical Publishing Company.

Novack J, Panow E, Tokarski J, Szafer W, and Stach J (1930) The second woolly rhinosceros (Coelodonta antiquitatis Blum.) from Starunia, Poland. *Bulletin de l'Academie Polonaise des Sciences et Lettres.* Ser. B Supplement: 1-7.

Painter TJ (1995) Chemical and microbiological aspects of the preservation process in Sphagnum Peat. RC Turner and RG Scaife (ed): *Bog Bodies: new discoveries and new perspectives.* London: British Museum press; 88-99.

Parry TJ and Pawsey RH (1990) *Principles of Microbiology for Students of Food Technology.* 2nd ed. Cheltenham: Stanley Thorne.

Peck WH (1998) Mummies of ancient Egypt. In A Cockburn, E Cockburn, and TA Reyman (eds.): *Mummies, Disease and Ancient Cultures.* 2nd ed. Cambridge University Press; 15-37.

Peng L (1995) Study of an ancient cadaver excavated from a Han Dynasty (207BC-AD220) tomb in Hunan Province. In *Proceedings of the World Congress on Mummy Studies* 2: 853-6. Santa Cruz de Tenerife: Museo Arqueologico Etnografico de Tenerife.

Pewe TL Rivard NR and Llano GA (1959) Mummified seal carcasses in the McMurdo Sound region, Antarctica. *Science* 130: 716.

Pike EC (2004) *The Disposition of 'Jimmy Garlick': some facts, fantasies and opinions regarding the history and future of the mummified man of St James's, Garlickhythe.* London: Church of St James Garlickhythe.

Rudenko SI (1970) *Frozen Tombs of Siberia: the Pazyrk Burials of Iron-age Horsemen.* London: Dent.

Spindler K (1994) T*he Man in the Ice, Volume 1: the preserved body of a Neolithic man reveals the secrets of the stone age.* London: Weidenfield & Nicolson.

Subrahmanyam M (1993) Storage of skin grafts in honey. *The Lancet* 341: 63-4.

Torre C and Cardellini C (1981) Ultrastructure of human tissues upon prolonged interment in metal-lined coffins. *Journal of Forensic Sciences* 26: 710-4.

Torre C, Zina AM, and Cardellini C (1982) The ultrastructure of corified skin. American *Journal of Forensic Medicine and Pathology* 3: 211-3.

Vreeland JM (1998) Mummies of Peru. In A Cockburn, E Cockburn, and TEA Reyman (eds.): *Mummmies, Disease and Ancient Culture,* 2nd edition; 154-189.

White WJ (1980) Frozen Tombs. *The London Archaeologist* 3: 274.

White WJ (1982) The mammoth in ice and snow: a reply to Ellenberger. *Kronos* 7: 62-66; *passim.*

White WJ (1985) Changing burial practice in late medieval England. J Petre (ed): *Richard III: Crown and People.* London: Yorkist History Trust; 371-9.

White WJ (1998) The excavation and study of human remains: a view from the floor. In M Cox (ed.): *Grave Concerns: Death and Burial in England 1700-1850.* York: CBA Research Report 113: 247-251.

White WJ (1999) The Iceman cometh. *Chemistry in Britain* 35: (7) July: 23.

Williams AC, Edwards HGM, and Barry BW (1999a) Iceman dispute. *Chemistry in Britain.* 35: (8) August: 20.

Williams AC, Edwards HGM, and Barry BW (1999b) Iceman issues. *Chemistry in Britain.* 35: (12) December: 23.

Willix DJ, Molan PC, and Harfoot CG (1992) A comparison of the sensitivity of wound-infecting species of bacteria to the antibacterial activity of manuka honey and other honey. *Journal of Applied Bacteriology* 73: 388-94.

Yamada TK, Kodou, T, and Takahashi-Iwanaga H (1990) Some 320-year-old soft tissue preserved by the presence of mercury. *Journal of Archaeological Science* 17: 383-392.

Yan F, McNally R, Kontanis EJ, and Sadik OA (2001) Preliminary quantitative investigation of post-mortem adipocere formation. *Journal of Forensic Sciences.* 46 (3): 609-14.

Zimmerman MR and Tedfold RH (1976) Histologic structures preserved for 21,300 years. Science 194: 183-4.

Selective Burial in Irish Megalithic Tombs:
Burial Practice, Age, Sex, and Representation in the Neolithic

Investigating Selective Burial Practices in the Irish Neolithic

Jessica F. Beckett

Darwin College, Silver Street, Cambridge, CB3 9EU, UK

Email: jfb40@cam.ac.uk

Abstract

Burial practice is a highly symbolic human activity through which concepts of the world are reflected in the representation and treatment of human remains. Through the integration of osteological analyses and social archaeological theory we may understand how societies used burial in socially significant ways. One such application is through the analysis of burial in megalithic monuments. Two important issues in regards to this analysis include the examination of how burials were used to manipulate, idealize, and distort the social situation rather than present direct reflections of the dead, and of the selective processes at such sites, in terms of status, sex, and age. However, we may ask how collective and multi-stage burials were selected for, and what, if any, criteria may have been used?

A case study of two Irish Neolithic chambered tombs is presented and the issue of selective burial is examined. The Poulnabrone and Parknabinnia tombs are located on the Burren, County Clare, Ireland, and date to the Early-Middle Neolithic period. A taphonomic study of the human skeletal remains was carried out in order to investigate burial practice. A representation of parts is presented to address the nature of primary and secondary burial, and possibly the circulation of remains. This examination of multi-stage burial is then used to contemplate the issue of selective burial processes, looking at the possibility of its occurrence, by which categories, and if not how the manipulation of remains in burial ritual may have served the living community.

Keywords Neolithic Ireland, Burren, megalithic tombs, burial practice, taphonomy

Introduction

Burial is a highly symbolic human activity through which concepts of the world are reflected in the representation and treatment of human remains. Through the integration of osteological analysis and social archaeological theory we may understand how societies used burial in socially significant ways. One such opportunity is through the analysis of burial ritual in megalithic monuments, and an important consideration is the categories for burial. Are the categories of age, sex, and status, as used for classification, valid, or does the process of collective, multi-stage burial distort our ideas of "selective processes"? What criteria were available to Neolithic peoples in selection for burial within these monuments, and can we access their systems of classification? These questions are examined in a case study of two Irish Neolithic chambered tombs located in County Clare. Through an osteological, taphonomic and theoretical analysis of the Poulnabrone portal tomb and the Parknabinnia chambered tomb deposits, we may begin to understand the complex and multi-stage processes of burial in megalithic monuments.

Background

The Burren is a geologically/ecologically unique area of Ireland. The barren and rocky terrain covers approximately 550 km^2, from the northwest of County Clare into southern Galway. Archaeological preservation is quite good, with over 500 monuments and features recorded (Jones, 1998a: 27). However, of 500 sites only 6 prehistoric sites have been excavated. There are some interesting regional peculiarities within the Burren. There appears to have been significant use of the area from the Early Neolithic (4,000BC). This period is dominated by ritual activity, represented by monuments/tombs, with no corresponding habitation sites found dating from this period. Given the number of preserved tombs, this may imply that people were living elsewhere or in temporary structures, possibly to the south of the Burren in more rich agricultural terrain. An increase in settlement and field systems began to take place into the later Neolithic and E.B.A. (Jones, 1997). The landscape is a unique upland region of limestone; this is a karstic landscape with exposed limestone plateaus (Feehan, 1992). While it is likely that Early Neolithic peoples assisted in the deforestation of Ireland beginning around 4,000 BC (Waddell, 1998:11), it is understood that both the glacial retreat and human interference contributed to the current landscape of the Burren (Feehan, 1992 and Waddell, 1992). Communities are likely to have used the area for grazing rather than for cultivation, as a pastoral economy were more predominant in the Early Neolithic (Cooney, 2000:44).

Distinct distributions of monument types occur across Ireland. Court tombs and portal tombs occur mostly in the north, passage tombs across the middle and north, and wedge tombs in the west (Waddell, 1998:57, 92-96). There is a great variety in tomb morphology on the Burren, with wedge tombs dominating the landscape (Jones and Gilmer, 1999). The heterogeneity dispels concepts of fixed locations for monuments, and the uniqueness of the Burren lies in the striking preservation of so many different types of monuments in one area, suggesting that this may have occurred in other places without the benefit of good preservation. The nature of the limestone landscape and materials used in building has surely preserved these sites. The patterns occurring upon the Burren might suggest that ideas as to tomb construction may have been borrowed from neighbouring groups within Ireland and adapted to fit this region's Neolithic communities.

Monuments

Two monuments from the Burren have been selected for study and will be discussed in relation to potential selective burial within Irish megalithic monuments/tombs. The two monuments included in the current study are the Parknabinnia chambered tomb and the Poulnabrone portal tomb.

Parknabinnia

Carleton Jones of NUI Galway excavated this site from 1998-2001. It is a simple chambered tomb, with some resemblance to court tombs. It has a rounded cairn, a narrow forecourt, and two chambers. It is unclear whether a roof existed, but, at the time of excavation, no roofing material was identified (Jones, 1998b; 1999). Recent Radiocarbon dating of the site reveals its use from c. 3,600 cal BC to 2,800 cal BC. Analysis of the remains, between 2000-2002, revealed approximately 19 individuals. Human bones, faunal bones, and a handful of typical Neolithic artefacts were placed continuously throughout the deposit (in the chambers and surrounding cairn). Unique patterning of bone in each context also existed with stone placed upon bone to seal each layer of the deposit. Remains were highly fragmented and mostly were disarticulated (except for a few cases of articulation) (Beckett, 2002).

Poulnabrone

Poulnabrone is a classic portal tomb, excavated from 1986-1988 by Anne Lynch (Lynch, 1994). It consists of a single chamber surrounded by three large stones, and covered in a large capstone. A small oval cairn potentially existed, although the presence of cairns for within these types of monuments is still debated

(Waddell, 1998:88). The excavation resulted in the recovery of Neolithic artefacts such as bone pendants, mushroom head pins, polished stone axes, stone beads, flint and chert scrapers, projectile points and plain pottery, faunal remains and human remains (Waddell, 1998:91). Approximately 22 individuals were represented at this monument and they appear to be similar to Parknabinnia's in terms of sex, age, diet and disease (ibid). The remains were unburnt and burnt, disarticulated, and heavily fragmented (Lynch, 1994; Lynch and O'Donnabháin, 1994). Radiocarbon dating revealed a span of 3800 to 3200 cal BC (Hedges et al., 1990). Morphologically the tomb differs from Parknabinnia as it has a single chamber, no forecourt, and is capped by a large stone. There is the possibility that Poulnabrone's remains were placed as a single deposition with more recent bones found stuffed into crevices below older ones (Cooney, 2000:96 and Lynch, 1994).

Examination and Discussion

The examination and discussion of these two sites is useful for several reasons. First, the monuments are located within 3 km of each other; they occur in depressions and are surrounded by Later Neolithic monuments. Secondly, they are morphologically different, but they have contemporaneous date ranges, and while this does not imply that they were in fact contemporary, their dates do overlap in certain instances. The pattern of human bones is similar in bioarchaeology and taphonomy. Some differences include the degree of fragmentation, the pattern of deposition, and the representation of parts of individuals, which may be due to the differences in the tombs themselves and their associated burial practices. It is possible that two distinct communities created similar monuments. On the other hand, a single community may have used these monuments with slightly different rites and purposes, but which fit within their entire cosmology/belief system.

The Act of Categorization in Irish Neolithic Burials

Burial in Irish megalithic monuments has often been described as involving "selective acts" (Cooney and Grogan, 1994, Waddell, 1998:91). It is inferred that individuals buried within these monuments were special to the community, because they were placed in "prominent" monuments. Archaeologists often impose the criteria of age, sex, and status to classify the selection that took place at these monuments. However, we must consider what categories of selection were available to an Irish Neolithic society. How does multi-stage and complex burial affect our understanding of these categories? Does the fact that the deposition sequence took place over several generations affect the understanding of ritual and categorization? Finally, the acts of burial must be considered in terms of the treatment, representation, and manipulation of remains within these monuments.

Before selection for burial takes place some system of classification for potential burial must exist. The relationship between classification and action has been described in two ways. The first, more static view, of this relationship derives from structural-functionalism and argues that human actions are guided by underlying unconscious structures (Renfrew and Bahn, 1996: 464, Kurzweil, 1980: 21). Structuralists, such as Lévi-Strauss, saw social interaction as the outward manifestation of cognitive structures (Layton, 1997:63). A familiar example derived from structural linguistics is binary opposition, which has been claimed to be a universal method of categorization (i.e. cooked/raw, left/right, dirty/clean) (Renfrew and Bahn, 1996: 464). In this context the structure has primacy over action (Giddens, 1984:2). This relationship between classification and action can also be explained in a less static way, such as through Bourdieu's theory of habitus (Bourdieu, 1989). Habitus are unconscious beliefs and processes of acquisition through experience that prefigure action (ibid: 83). They are socially constituted abstract principles held about the nature of reality, which are then implemented in action. Habitus is situational and a product of historical practices (Bourdieu, 1989:82-83), but, is improvisation rather than predetermined rules (Layton, 1997:204), so knowledge is produced and reproduced, with limitless options for action, even if the choices themselves are not unlimited.

It is clear that all humans, past and present, classify their worlds. Lévi-Strauss (1966) argued that it is a universal drive to order the world by schemes of classification. However, it may be slightly presumptuous to declare that a past system or scheme of classification can be understood fully. Yet, this is not to deny any attempt to understand those systems. If actions are carried out under the guidance of unconscious beliefs or knowledge, inherent structures in our mind, or purposeful manipulations, then these actions should create patterns, which can be accessed, in the material evidence. While it may be difficult to completely explain the purpose behind those patterns, it is never the less a valuable pursuit, particularly in mortuary studies.

Acts of burial themselves reveal a relationship between classification and action in the selection for burial. This action requires a system of classification which guides the actor in terms of who is buried, how are they buried, and where are they buried. It can be inferred that the relationship between classifying things and taking action upon that system is reflexive. On the one hand, there are rules (dictated by culture or society), which govern proper burial treatment, and in the same instance categories may be reconstructed through action, which can justify or legitimate a view or position within society. In this way rules may possibly be changed or reclassified as needed. When Neolithic peoples selected for burial they were perhaps constructing and reconstructing the chosen categories through their actions, and those actions are revealed in the burial evidence. These practices were organized and patterned. Burial in megalithic monuments was complex and suggests intentional acts of burial, which were well thought out and governed by existing or created rules. Is there evidence that bodies were selected for based upon age, sex or status at these monuments or is this a bias placed upon the evidence by archaeologists? A consideration of some theoretical arguments and the burial evidence is necessary to better understand these questions.

Theoretical arguments; supporting the bone evidence?

The bone evidence from Poulnabrone and Parknabinnia reveal that some system of classification and or selection was taking place at these monuments, and through an examination of this evidence, it may be possible to identify how burials were selected for. Firstly, it was found that most of the bone was in a disarticulated state at both sites. Only five articulations were found at Poulnabrone, including vertebrae and phalanges (Table 1), while 46 specific articulations and bone groupings were identified at Parknabinnia (Table 1). At Parknabinnia there was one case of an articulated pelvis and femur, articulated vertebrae, tarsals, metatarsals, carpals and metacarpals (Beckett, 2002). The primary rite at both sites was inhumation. Eighty-three burnt human bones and 792 unidentified burnt bones were found at Poulnabrone. The majority of these were burnt blue/black, 91%, which indicates scorching rather than cremation (Buikstra and Ubelaker, 1994: 96). At Parknabinnia 105 burnt human bones were identified, with 2,775 unidentified burnt items, including bone and charcoal. The majority of these burnt items were warped, white in colour, and had longitudinal cracking across the bone. These indicate burning at very high temperatures such as in cremation (ibid: 95). The presence of many small pieces of burnt bone and charcoal also suggest that material from pyres was collected and placed into this tomb.

Table 1: A comparison of bone from Poulnabrone and Parknabinnia

	Poulnabrone	**Parknabinnia**
Total Bone	14,936	20,750
Human Bone	4,755	6,146
Unidentified Bone	10,181	14,604
MNI	22	19
Articulated bones	5	46
Disarticulated bones	14,931	20,704
Burnt Human	83	105
Burnt Unidentified	792	2,775
Adults % of MNI	64%	78%
Subadults % of MNI	36%	21%
Sexed Males	4	2
Sexed Females	4	5

Collective versus individual burial

Collective rites predominate over individual burial at most Irish megalithic monuments (Waddell, 1998). The collective burials are generally disarticulated, and in mixed states, suggesting secondary burial (Herity, 1987:159). However, the understanding of Irish burial rites is very limited. This is due to the fact that very few remains have been recovered from monuments within Ireland, the total being some 400 individuals (Cooney, 1992), and yet there are over 1500 monuments recorded in Ireland (Waddell, 1998). Thus our knowledge about typical Neolithic burial patterns is somewhat skewed by the small amount of remains found and the types of burial rites associated with their burial.

Cremation versus inhumation

Cremation is considered to be more common than inhumation in terms of burial rites in Irish megalithic tombs, particularly in passage tombs, wedge tombs, and court tombs (Waddell, 1998, Herity, 1987). Cooney (2000:68) also notes the possibility that differential treatment between cremation and inhumation existed based upon age as well. Yet, this is not the case at Poulnabrone and Parknabinnia. Both adults and children were interred unburnt and burnt. The limited number of burial finds in Ireland indeed limits a full understanding of these rites.

Age

Of 400 burials from megalithic contexts in Ireland, 68% are of adults and 32% are of children (Cooney and Grogan, 1994:70). This is not an accurate representation of a living Neolithic population, given likely higher infant mortality at this time (ibid: 70; Burgess, 1980:162). What proportion of the Neolithic population consisted of children? It has been proposed that at least half of the living population of the Neolithic would have been children (Cooney, 2000:126).

However, these Early Neolithic Irish populations were not under the same pressures as intensive agricultural societies, and may have had a better overall living standard and lower infant mortality rate. Depending upon the infant mortality rates over this period, 30% of remains found being those of subadults is a relatively high percentage of children recovered. As children's remains are more fragile than adult remains (Henderson, 1987: 45), fewer representations of children are likely to be preserved. They are more susceptible to erosion processes, and small remains may also be subjected to biases both in the reworking of deposits and later recovery processes. This implies that age is not a selection basis for inclusion in megalithic tombs.

Subadult remains at Poulnabrone and Parknabinnia account for 32% and 22% of the individuals identified at each site. Children were not categorically excluded. Considering that adult remains are highly fragmented, it is surprising that children's remains were recovered at all

as they are more susceptible to destruction. We can conclude that age does not seem to be a factor in selection for deposition within the tombs.

Sex

Was there categorization based on biological sex? Representations of female and male remains are found in most Irish collective monuments (Cooney 1992:129). Both at Poulnabrone and Parknabinnia, male and female remains are represented as well. Poulnabrone had approximately equal representation of males and females (eight adult remains were sexed, with four of each) (Lynch, 1994:18). At Parknabinnia 60 bones were assessed for sex using qualitative visual observations of the skull and pelvis, and metric measurements of the long bones, with 16 scored as ambiguous, 16 male, and 28 female. Of these 60 bones, however, only a few overlap in each category. Skulls show an MNI of two, with one possible female and one ambiguous. Pelves indicate at least five individuals with two males, two ambiguous, and one female. However, the measurements taken on the long bones show at least seven individuals with five females and two males. Those sexed remains certainly do not represent the total number of adults counted for, however. Due to the high degree of fragmentation most of the remains cannot be sexed. Thus, while there seem to be more females than males, we cannot conclusively say that this was a factor in selection at this site.

Status

Next the question of status can be addressed based upon those arguments put forth by Bindord (1971) in "Mortuary Practices; their study and potential." Binford (1971: 20-21) identified dimensional distinctions among four types of subsistence categories, and noted three variables of distinction found in treatment of the body, preparation of the facility, and grave furniture. His argument assumes that status in life carries through into death, or is directly mirrored in death, and that those who bury the dead translate this status into these categories. This was validated by the assertion that treatment of the dead was related to the social position the deceased held in life and that burial practices were influenced by social organization (Wason, 1994: 67).

However, Parker-Pearson (2001: 32) argues that burial events allow social roles to be manipulated, acquired, and discarded. This is particularly important in collective burials. In these cases it may be more worthwhile to view burial as an indirect reflection of the social situation because it is affected by ideology, cosmology, and symbolism. In other words, it is the living that buries the dead, and it is the living that holds ideas (structures if you will) of how best to represent the dead in death. In this manner the dead may be manipulated to promote living people's social situation; while the individual may not have been rich in life, placing valuable items into their grave may actually promote their descendant's social positions. The dead may also be idealized in death, or used to distort the social situation for ideological purposes.

Were megalithic monuments regarded as "high status" places, where only special, or high status individuals were buried? Cooney (2000: 96) argues that, because of the disparity in age ratios, and the number of individuals recovered from Neolithic tombs, that these tombs were not the burial locations for the entire population, and were instead probably used for the interment of special individuals. Waddell (1998: 85, 91) concurs that there was not full and formal burial of all members of the community in megalithic monuments, and that age and sex profiles indicate selection of specific individuals for this "special privilege" of megalithic tomb burial. It is important to remember, though, that the number of individuals recovered from megalithic monuments most probably represent only a small proportion of those originally buried in the tombs. Counts of MNI, therefore, should be scrutinized as the methodology for estimating the number of individuals may not be entirely applicable to megalithic monuments with collective burial, changing functions, and behaviours change over time.

The locations of the monuments, although sometimes set apart from habitation sites, they also formed part of everyday life (Cooney, 2000: 23). While monuments may have been permanent fixtures in the landscape they were not unchanging. Sites had histories prior to the construction of monuments, and the purpose of these monuments altered over the course of generations (ibid: 125). Many monuments were blocked and sealed; some continued to be used for other purposes, others were reused generations later (ibid: 125).

Monuments also had varying levels of access to the population; some remained open to the entire community, while others were closed and held secret (Bradley, 1998: 62). Construction of monuments would have varied as well, with some requiring large amounts of effort by the entire community and others by only a few individuals (Renfrew, 1983). Furthermore, it is difficult to point to a single function of megalithic monuments as well and it is possible that they served as territorial markers, places for the disposal of the dead, signalling systems, shrines, or even conversion techniques (Renfrew, 1983; Ashbee, 1978, Chapman, 1981; Fleming, 1973; Case, 1973; Sherratt, 1995; Bradley, 1998; Atkinson, 1968; Kinnes, 1975). There is much variation in the record between monuments in place and time.

If monuments were high status places, then should we expect the social organization of Neolithic societies to include ranking, division of labour, or even specialists? Social organization at this time probably consisted of segmentary societies, kin based, with small villages or even temporary habitations (Cooney, 2000: 5). It is clear that many types of social groupings probably were in existence during the Neolithic. In terms of divisions or ranking it was probably in the world of ritual and

religion, where certain individuals (perhaps elders) served as part-time religious specialists. Renfrew (1983: 14) says of his work at Quanterness in Orkney, that there was equal access to that tomb and a balanced representation of ages and sexes with no ranking. He interprets this monument as being the work of a corporate group of a segmentary society made up of approximately 50-100 people (ibid: 12).

A status bound interpretation requires assumptions that social distinctions are mirrored in the treatment of the dead. Yet, burial events are likely to have been manipulated so that roles may be emphasized, exaggerated, acquired or discarded. Status implies social division within society, and while Neolithic societies may not have been egalitarian, they may have masked existing social distinctions either in the use of burial objects placed with the dead or in burial practices. Thus, burial patterns may not represent true mortality rates or social facts.

The distinction of grave goods, however, also falls short in identifying status. Irish megalithic monuments generally possess little artefactual evidence. For instance, court tombs, portal tombs and wedge tombs all include everyday use items, such as Neolithic pottery (usually fragmented), stone tools and beads (Waddell, 1998: 57-92). Only in passage tombs do we find evidence of more ritualized or specialized artefacts (ibid: 73). It appears that artefacts are not associated with "individuals" at Poulnabrone or Parknabinnia and thus it may be more useful to view these items as offerings. Status, therefore, seems an invalid category for selection within megalithic monuments.

Evidence of burials at Poulnabrone and Parknabinnia

The evidence for burial reveals complex rites and practices occurred at Poulnabrone and Parknabinnia. Using taphonomic methods, the bone material from both sites was analyzed according to degree of fragmentation, type of fragmentation, completeness, articulations, the presence of burning, and for environmental/physical evidence such as weathering and dissolution, abrasions, polishing, root markings, accretions and whether there were further modifications made to the bones either by humans or animals. At Poulnabrone there was a large amount of fragmentation identified. Most of these fragments were highly weathered, cracked and split, and 87% were less than half complete (Table 2). A representation of parts was also carried out, which calculates the percent of expected bones that should be found for each element, if whole bodies were interred and recovered, by taking the amount of bones found for an individual element divided by the expected and times 100 to reveal the percent of representation. In the case of Poulnabrone there should be 22 skulls, 528 vertebrae and 264 long bones if these individuals were placed into the tomb complete.

Table 2. A comparison of taphonomy from Poulnabrone and Parknabinnia

	Poulnabrone	Parknabinnia
% bone < 5 cm	90%	90%
% bone < ½ complete	87%	94%
Weathering	93%	95.5%
No weathering	7%	4.5%
Plant/root etching	21%	1%
Polish/Abrasion	<1%	<1%
Insect Marks	<1%	.1%
Accretions (calcium/fungus)	.5%	.7%

However, natural and cultural factors were at work over the last 6,000 years, and so all of the parts are not represented. The representation of body parts reveals that there are under-representations of skulls, vertebrae, humeri and radii, pelvis, sacrum, coccyx and lower long bones (Figures 1 and 2). However, looking at the figures for adult bones, there is a notable difference between the scapulae and humeri (91% versus 56%) and the upper long bones and carpals (scaphoids = 94% representation) (Figures 3 and 4). Generally speaking hands and feet are less represented in burial situations because they are subject to excavator bias (small parts go missing) and are more susceptible to degradation (Waldron, 1987). However, there should be at least the same amount of carpals and metacarpals as upper long bones, yet the reverse is true. A notable difference can also be found between the femur and patella (31% versus 88%). There is also higher representation of parts for tarsals versus the lower long bones, and in particular an unusual amount of naviculars (78%). In terms of deposition there were also bones with a later Radiocarbon date below ones with earlier Radiocarbon dates and placed down into grykes, or crevices in the limestone bedrock (Cooney 2000: 96). This would suggest a mixing of the strata whereby older bones came to rest on top of younger ones. Possible explanations are that the remains from Poulnabrone were collected elsewhere and placed into the chamber later, or that collections of these missing items were made from this site and taken elsewhere. Poulnabrone most probably represents secondary burial rites. Deliberate disturbance and circulation of bones during the Irish Neolithic has been considered (Cooney and Grogan, 1994: 70) and may be likely at either Poulnabrone or Parknabinnia.

More fragments were found at Parknabinnia; bones were also slightly less complete than at Poulnabrone (Table 2). The taphonomy was quite similar, in that the bones were weathered, with thinning of the exterior layers of bone, calcium and fungus accretions, and fewer plant markings. There were no animal marks and only one possible cutmark, but it is unclear if this was faunal. The representation of body parts reveals less striking patterns between long bones and hand and feet (Figures 1 and 2).

However, there were under-representations of vertebrae, carpals, ribs, coccyx, and foot phalanges. With the adult remains, there is a notable difference between skulls and the atlas and axis vertebrae (47% v. 80% v. 100%) (Figures 3 and 4). Metatarsals are under-represented but the tarsals occur roughly on an equal basis with the lower long bones.

Most fragile and small bones are underrepresented which is not unusual given their potential loss in transition or excavation and their susceptibility to degradation. The contextual evidence, such as the placement of groups of bone and articulated parts under rock suggests much reworking of the deposit, as does the condition and fragmentation of the parts. A study of refits may help to clarify the burial practices at this sight. Both natural and cultural factors have effected the nature and condition of bones here and it is possible that secondary burial rites were occurring at this sight as well, however, the evidence points to inhumation with successive depositions where bodies were possible placed into the tomb mostly complete, left to decompose and then attended to later when successive interments were made.

It is clear that burial was patterned within megalithic monuments. Some Irish megalithic sites exhibit a preference for skulls and long bones (Cooney and Grogan, 1994: 68). Body symmetry and bone selection may well have been a factor in representation of remains within tombs (Shanks and Tilley, 1982: 150). Treatment may have included excarnation to access skeletal parts (Renfrew, 1979). If secondary burial rites occurred, then it can be inferred that bodies were treated elsewhere before insertion. No evidence was found of manipulative defleshing, or excarnation at either Parknabinnia or Poulnabrone. No cut marks were present and no evidence of animal gnawing was found, either of which might have indicated that bodies were exposed prior to burial. There still seems to be some distinction between fleshed and unfleshed parts with unusual deposition and pattern of remains. Bones could have represented whole bodies in the same manner as individuals represented the community.

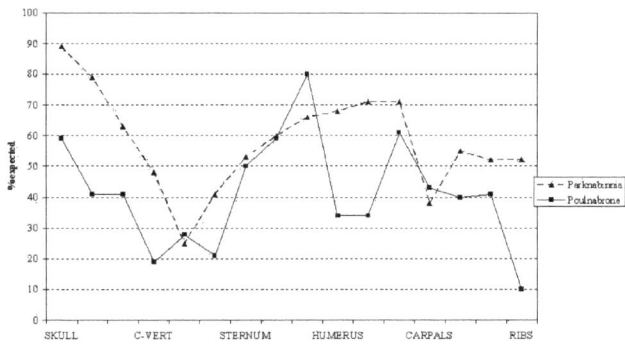

Figure 1. Representation of Upper Body Parts, All Individuals Compared

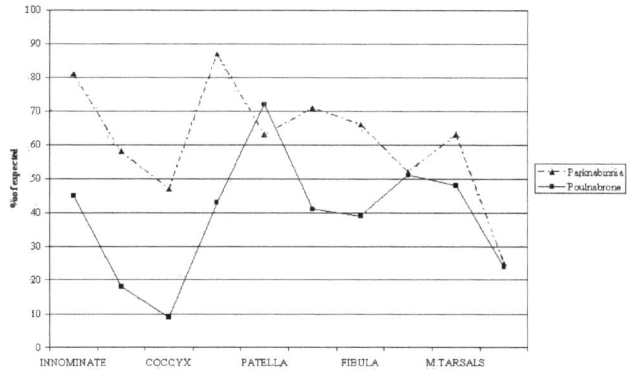

Figure 2. Representation of Lower Body Parts, All Individuals Compared

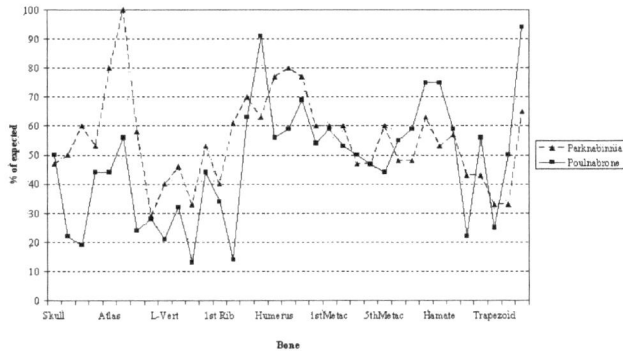

Figure 3. Representation of Upper Body Parts, Adults Compared

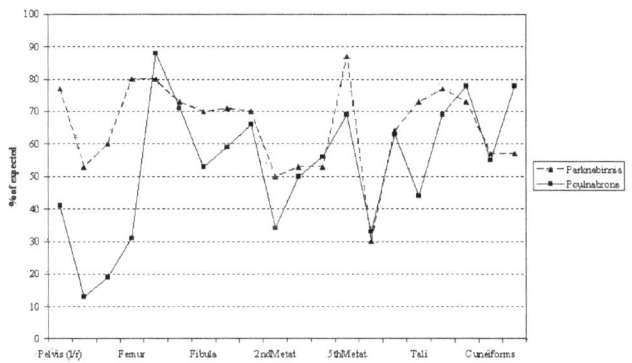

Figure 4. Representation of Lower Body Parts, Adults Compared

Burial Patterning and Theoretically Useful Categories

Selection based upon age, sex, or status is too simple to fully understand burial practice in megalithic monuments in Ireland. At either Parknabinnia or Poulnabrone these categories are not clearly defined or distinguished. Instead, the following categories in action have been demonstrated:

1. Collective over individual burial

2. Inhumation versus cremation

3. Bones versus flesh

4. Secondary versus primary burial

5. Body part representation

What can be inferred about this Neolithic society through their categorization of burial in these ways? How were the dead represented through burial and how do the actions of the living toward the dead relate to the potential use of burials and burial locations? Communal versus individual identity was emphasized during the Neolithic at both these sites. There were patterned, intentional, and symbolic behaviours played out in the practice of interring multiple bodies or parts of bodies. It is possible that the use of the bodies as symbolic vehicles represents a society's social construction of reality and may have acted to assert the collective nature of that society over the individual (Shanks and Tilley, 1982: 134, 150). This may have been an exaggerated form of communal existence, with burial then reflecting an idealized form of the community (Cooney, 1992: 140-141). The efforts to represent the dead in this manner can demonstrate a strong tie to the ancestors, by creating lasting connections with the world of the dead and revealing continuity and the importance of the ancestors for the living (Cooney, 2000: 90 and Hodder, 1990: 25).

The opposition found between flesh and bone also reveals how substances were viewed for burial. By selecting bone items, the population may have been symbolically recreating the whole body. The patterns of deposition, taphonomy and representations of parts at Poulnabrone, in particular, suggest individual bones, rather than articulated items or whole bodies, were selected. In order to access bones in this way, bodies must have been at least partially decomposed.

It is likely that the manipulation of bodies occurred within an ideological framework. The living community were perhaps representing the dead as an ancestral community and treating them in a manner that was consistent with their belief system, including secondary burial, body part selection, and circulation of bones. As has been shown, Poulnabrone represents both secondary burial and body part selection. With a high fragmentation rate and the preferential presence of certain body parts the collection has been shown to be highly disturbed and it is possible that bones were collected from other monuments for insertion within the Poulnabrone tomb. Parknabinnia, on the other hand, may show efforts to collect particular bones (possibly skulls) from monument for deposition elsewhere. The sealing of layers by rock may also suggest that bone was "cleaned up" before successive interments. This would explain why partially articulated parts are found as well as the presence of more bones to the north and south of the chamber. The population was acting upon bodies in order to transform them into the world of the dead, creating a tie between the living and the dead, and thereby the tomb may also have symbolized a vehicle of remembrance.

Conclusion

An analysis of the methods for categorization is an effective way of treating the evidence for human burial in megalithic monuments. It needs to be made aware how categories were reconstructed in action, the intentions of categorization, and how categories are reflected in action and vice versa. Megalithic burial was a sequence of categorical acts of reclassification. Neolithic peoples categorized their world and in turn created categories and meaning through their actions. Burials were highly organized, patterned, and representative of worldviews and ideological systems.

However, care should be taken when making classifications through archaeological analyses. The complexity of the burial rite, differential burial, reuse and manipulation of funerary deposits, and limits within modern methodologies complicates the identification of prehistoric categories. Issues such as counts of MNI within such complex monuments and the length of use of monuments also restrict an accurate view of how many people were buried in these monuments and whether particular categories were in use for hundreds of years and several generations. It cannot be assumed that categories were unchanging or that burial rites were consistent over the use/reuse period of a monument.

Selection would have taken place based upon some cultural system of categorization, but there may be biases in the sample and in the views created about these categories. This does not negate the potential use in identifying categories, but should be recognized as a hindrance in interpretation. Some recognition of the difference in burial attitude may also be possible with a closer analysis of the sequence of burial, refits studies, GIS, and further dating of materials within the deposits. This case study has hopefully allowed some recognition of the benefits of identifying categories and their meaning within Neolithic burial and a tentative interpretation of the categories employed by these societies has proved possible.

Acknowledgements

The author would like to thank the Gates Cambridge Trust, Darwin College, and the Department of Archaeology (University of Cambridge) for funding the current research.

Literature Cited

Ashbee P. 1978. *The ancient British: a social-archaeological narrative*. Geo Books: Norwich.

Atkinson RJC. 1968. Old mortality: some aspects of burial and population in Neolithic England. In *Studies in Ancient Europe: essays presented to Stuart Piggott*, Coles JM and Simpson DDA (eds.). University of Leicester Press: Leicester; 83-93

Beckett J. 2002. *An Analysis of the Parknabinnia Chambered Tomb; County Clare, Ireland; Ideology and Ritual during the Early Neolithic*. Unpublished Masters Thesis, San Diego State University: San Diego.

Binford L. 1971. Mortuary practices their study and potential. In *Approaches to the Social Dimensions of Mortuary Practices*, Brown J (ed.). Memoirs of the Society for American Archaeology 25.

Bourdieu P. 1989. *Outline of a Theory of Practice*. Translated Nice R. Cambridge University Press: Cambridge.

Bradley R. 1998. *The Significance of Monuments: On the Shaping of Human Experience in Neolithic and Bronze Age Europe*. Routledge: London.

Burgess C. 1980. *The Age of Stonehenge*. Dent: London.

Case H. 1973. A ritual site in Northeast Ireland. In *Megalithic Graves and Ritual*, Daniel G and Kjaerum P (eds.). Jutland Archaeological Society: Copenhagen.

Chapman RW. 1981. Emergence of formal disposal areas and the "problem" of megalithic tombs in prehistoric Europe. In *Prehistoric Europe*, Chapman RW, Kinnes I and Randsborg K (eds.). Cambridge University Press: Cambridge; 71-82.

Cooney G. 1992. Body Politics and Grave Messages: Irish Neolithic Mortuary Practices. In *Vessels for the Ancestors,* Sharples N and Sheridan A (eds.). Edinburgh University Press: Edinburgh: 128-142.

Cooney G. 2000. *Landscapes of Neolithic Ireland*. Routledge: London.

Cooney G. and Grogan E. 1994. Irish Prehistory: a social perspective. Wordwell, Ltd: Dublin.

Feehan J. 1992. The Rocks and Landforms of the Burren. In *The Book of the Burren*, O'Connell JW and Korff A (eds.). Tír Eolas: Galway; 14-23.

Fleming A. 1973. Tombs for the Living. *Man* VIII 177-93.

Giddens A. 1984. *The Constitution of Society*. Polity Press: Cambridge.

Herity M. 1987. The Finds from Irish Court Tombs. *Proceedings of the Royal Irish Academy* 87C(5): 104-281.

Hedges REM, Housley RA, Law IA, and Bronk CR. 1990. Radiocarbon dates from the Oxford AMS system. *Archaeometry* 32: 101-8.

Henderson J. 1987. Factors determining the state of preservation of human remains. In *Death, Decay, and Reconstruction*, Boddington A, Garland AN, and Janaway R. (eds.). Manchester University Press: Manchester; 43-54.

Hodder I. 1990. *The Domestication of Europe*. Blackwell Publishers Inc: Oxford.

Jones C. 1998a. The Discovery and Dating of the Prehistoric Landscape of Roughan Hill in Co. Clare. *The Journal of Irish Archaeology* 9: 27-43.

Jones C. 1998b. *Interim report on the first season of excavation at Clare 153, a court tomb in Parknabinnia, Kilnaboy, County Clare.* Submitted to the National Museum of Ireland, License #98E0230.

Jones C. 1999. *Interim report on the second season of excavation at Clare 153, a court tomb in Parknabinnia, Kilnaboy, County Clare.* Submitted to the National Museum of Ireland, License #98E0230.

Jones C. and Gilmer A. 1999. Roughan Hill, a Final Neolithic/Early Bronze Age landscape revealed. *Archaeology Ireland* Spring 1999: 30-32.

Kinnes I. 1975. Monumental Function in British Neolithic Burial Practices. *World Archaeology* VII: 16-29.

Kurzweil E. 1980. *The Age of Structuralism*. Columbia University Press: New York.

Layton R. 1997. *An Introduction to theory in anthropology.* Cambridge University Press: Cambridge.

Lévi-Strauss C. 1966. *The Savage Mind.* Penguin Books, Ltd: New York.

Lynch A. 1994. Poulnabrone portal tomb. Burren, Co. Clare, *Irish Association for Quaternary Studies Field Guide* 18: 18-20.

Lynch A. and O'Donnabháin B. 1994. Poulnabrone, Co. Clare. *The Other Clare* 18: 5-7.

Parker-Pearson M. 2001. *The Archaeology of Death and Burial.* Texas A&M University Press: College Station.

Renfrew AC. 1979. *Investigations in Orkney.* Society of Antiquaries: London.

Renfrew AC. 1983. Introduction: The Megalith Builders of Western Europe. In *The Megalithic Monuments of Western Europe: the latest evidence presented by nine leading authorities*, Renfrew AC (ed.). Thames and Hudson: London; 8-17.

Renfrew AC. and Bahn P. 1996. *Archaeology: Theory, Method and Practice.* Thames and Hudson: London.

Shanks M and Tilley C. 1982. Ideology, Symbolic power and ritual communication: reinterpretations of Neolithic mortuary practices. In *Symbolic and Structural Archaeology,* Hodder I (ed.). Cambridge University Press: Cambridge; 129-154.

Sherratt A. 1995. Instruments of Conversion? The role of megaliths in the Mesolithic/ Neolithic transition in North Western Europe. In *Oxford Journal of Archaeology* 14: 245-60.

Waddell J. 1992. The First People; The Prehistoric Burren. In *The Book of the Burren*, O'Connell, JW and Korff A (eds.). Tír Eolas: Galway; 59-76.

Waddell J. 1998. *The Prehistoric Archaeology of Ireland.* Galway University Press: Galway.

Waldron T. 1987. The Relative Survival of the Human Skeleton: Implications for Palaeopathology. In *Death, Decay, and Reconstruction*, Boddington A, Garland AN, and Janaway R. (eds.). Manchester University Press: Manchester; 55-64.

Wason PK. 1994. *The Archaeology of Rank.* Cambridge University Press: Cambridge.

Disturbing the dead: the displacement and destruction of skeletal remains in early medieval Wessex, c.600-1100AD.

Disturbing the dead

Annia Kristina Cherryson

Department of Archaeology, University of Sheffield, Northgate House, West Street, Sheffield S1 4ET

e-mail address for correspondence: a.k.cherryson@sheffield.ac.uk

Abstract: For over a millennium, the skeletal remains of those laid to rest in England's churchyards were often disturbed and destroyed by the bodies of later generations or by ecclesiastical and secular buildings. This study examines the levels of post-burial disturbance seen in Wessex during the early medieval period, c. 600-1100AD, a period which saw the advent of churchyard burial in England. The evidence for post-burial disturbance of the deceased has been assessed in 21 early medieval cemeteries from Wessex. This revealed a general trend of higher levels of grave disturbance in churchyards when compared to the field cemeteries that both preceded and co-existed with the churchyards. Much of the skeletal disturbance when present in earlier field cemeteries can best be characterised as the reuse of pre-existing graves while that found in the later churchyard cemeteries was primarily the result of the intercutting by later graves. The later churchyards also saw the deposition of displaced skeletal remains in charnel pits and the use of displaced skulls as "pillow stones" for other burials. These higher levels of post-burial disturbance seen in the later Saxon churchyards appear to be the product of the advent of churchyard burial and the increasing influence of the church over burial. However, these changes in the post-burial treatment of the deceased should also be seen, in part, as a practical response to the processes of urbanisation during the late Saxon period.

Keywords — post-burial disturbance, early medieval Wessex, churchyards.

Introduction

"May they rest in peace" is often said of the dead, but, in truth, the reality is very different. For the vast majority of those laid to rest in churchyards over the last millennium, this was often not the case, with their mortal remains disturbed, displaced or destroyed by the burials of later generations or by buildings (either ecclesiastical or secular). This paper examines the evidence for the post-burial treatment of the deceased during the early medieval period, a period which saw the origins of churchyard burial. In particular, it seeks to examine the extent to which the level and nature of post-burial disturbance seen in the churchyards of this period differs from that seen in the field cemeteries of the seventh and eighth century, which both preceding and co-existed with them. The factors which may have contributed to the level of post-burial disturbance of the deceased seen in the churchyards of the early medieval period are then considered.

The evidence for the post-burial treatment of the deceased from early medieval Wessex

The level of post-burial disturbance was examined in 21 early medieval cemeteries from Wessex (see figure 1 for

locations and table 1 for a summary of the information for each site). Thirteen of these sites were field cemeteries, not associated with any ecclesiastical buildings. Of the thirteen, eleven were rural burial grounds founded during the late sixth and seventh centuries and were usually short-lived, with ten of the eleven going out of use by or during the eighth century. There is one slightly atypical cemetery among these eleven sites, the long-lived burial ground of Bevis Grave (Hants) (Rudkin 2001), which, although founded in the seventh century, continued in use until the tenth. Bevis Grave, with over 80 individuals, is also larger than the other field cemeteries, which tended to be small with the number of burials ranging from 15 to 60. The final two field cemeteries included within the study, differed from the others in that they were later foundations. One was the small cemetery at Cook Street, Hants, which was in use during the eighth century and lay within the middle Saxon emporium of Hamwic (Garner 1993;2001, Garner & Vincent 1997). The other burial ground, associated with a manorial estate at Portchester (Hants) dates to the eleventh century (Cunliffe 1976).

The other eight cemeteries within this study are either known or strongly suspected to be associated with churches (table 1 and figure 1) and are examples of the early medieval churchyards, which gradually replaced the field cemeteries from the seventh century onwards.

Table 1: The level and nature of post-burial disturbance seen in early medieval cemeteries in Wessex.

Site	Date of site	Type of site	No. of burials[1]	Ecclesiastical buildings	Level of post burial disturbance	Nature of disturbance[2]	References
Bargates (Do)	Late 6th-7th century	Rural	30	No	None – but no bone survives	None of graves intercut	Jarvis 1983
Winnall II (Ha)	7th century	Rural	47	No	None	-	Meaney & Hawkes 1970
Monkton Deverill (Wi)	c. 7th century	Rural	15	No	None	-	Rawlings 1995
Portsdown II (Ha)	7th century	Rural	21	No	Low-moderature	Re-use of 2 graves	Corney 1967
Snell's Corner (Ha)	7th century	Rural	33	No	None	-	Knocker 1955
Ulwell (Do)	7th century	Rural	55	No	Low-moderate	Re-use & intercutting of graves	Cox 1989
Bevis Grave (Ha)	7th-10th century	Rural	88	No	Low-moderate	Re-use of 11 graves, intercutting of three graves.	Rudkin 2001
Didcot (Ox)	7th century	Rural	17	No	None	-	Boyle et al 1995
Burghclere (Bk)	7th century	Rural		No	None- but no bone survives	No intercutting of graves	Butterworth & Lobb 1992
SOU 862 (Ha)		Rural	16	No	None	-	Southern Archaeological Services 1998.
St. Mary's Stadium (Ha)	Late 7th early 8th century	Rural	23	No	Low-Moderate	8 graves disturbed by later middle Saxon pits	Birbeck & Smith 2003
Beckery Chapel (So)	Middle Saxon	Monastic	58	Timber chapel or tomb shrine	Low	Number of burials disturbed by construction of late Saxon/Norman chapel II or later chapel III	Rahtz & Hirst 1974
SOU 13 (Ha)	8th-9th century	Urban	81	Timber church	High	Approximately 1/3 of bodies redeposited, many others loss parts of body to later burials	Morton 1992a
Cook Street (Ha)	Early 8th century	Urban	21	No	Low	1 intercut burial	Garner 1993, 2001; Garner & Vincent 1997
Staple Gardens (Ha)	Mid 9th-11th century	Urban	288	Church suspected	Moderate-high	Intercutting burials	Kipling & Scobie 1990
Bath Abbey (So)	Late Saxon	Urban	31	Abbey church	Low	1 intercut burial & charnel pit from construction of Norman abbey	Bell 1996
Barnstaple (Dv)	Late Saxon	Urban	105	Church suspected	Moderate	Intercutting of graves & a few burials disturbed by construction of moat of Norman castle	Miles 1984
Exeter Cathedral (Dv)	Middle-late Saxon	Urban	114	Minster church	Moderate-high	Intercutting burials & some burials disturbed by construction work	Henderson & Bidwell 1982
Wells Cathedral (So)	Middle-late Saxon	Urban	242	Minster church/ Cathedral	Moderate	Intercutting burials & graves disturbed by later buildings.	Rodwell 2001
Trowbridge (Wi)	10th-early 12th century	Manorial	164	Church	Moderate	Intercutting rows of burials, with later rows disturbing earlier burials.	Graham & Davies 1993
Portchester (Ha)	11th century	Manorial?	22	No	Low	1 example of an intercut grave, but no disturbance of any bones & reburial of 2 individuals, possibly disturbed by building work.	Cunliffe 1976

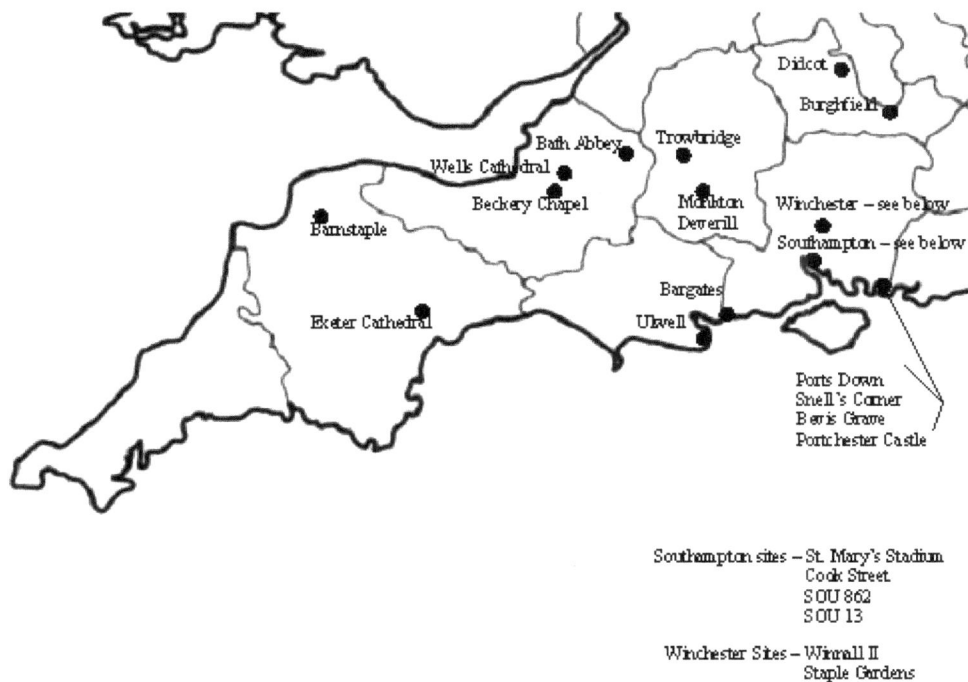

Figure 1. Location of cemeteries used in study

Unlike the majority of the field cemeteries that they superseded, many of the churchyards were long lived with burial at Wells Cathedral (Somset) (Rodwell 2001), Exeter Cathedral (Devon) (Henderson & Bidwell 1982), Bath Abbey (Somset) (Bell 1996) and Trowbridge, (Wilts) (Graham & Davies 1993) continuing throughout the late Saxon period, and beyond, into the medieval or post-medieval periods. As such, unlike the earlier field cemeteries, many churchyards contain larger numbers of inhumations, and this is reflected within this study, with five of the eight churchyards containing the remains of more than a hundred individuals, despite being only partially excavated. Six of the churchyards lie within urban centres, while the manorial churchyard at Trowbridge (Graham & Davies 1993) and the monastic cemetery associated with Beckery Chapel (Somset) (Rahtz & Hirst 1974) lie within rural contexts.

Variations in the quality of recording and the differences in the degree of post-eleventh-century disturbance between sites, made it difficult to quantify the levels of post-burial disturbance in the cemeteries. As such, a descriptive system was developed which categorised the levels of disturbance as none, low, moderate and high to allow qualitative comparisons between cemeteries (as shown below):

- None-No evidence of post-burial disturbance of the deceased.

- Low-Evidence for intercutting or re-use seen in only 1 or 2 graves.

- Moderate -Evidence for intercutting or re-use observed in a few graves.

- High-Widespread evidence of the post-burial disturbance of the deceased.

Variations in levels of post burial disturbance among cemeteries within the study

The levels of post-burial disturbance observed in the 21 sites within the study are given in table 1. There were significant differences seen in the levels of post-burial disturbance in field cemeteries when compared with the churchyard cemeteries. In general, lower levels of post-burial disturbance were observed in the thirteen field cemeteries. No evidence for any post-burial disturbance of early medieval date was observed in seven field cemeteries, Bargates (Dorset) (Jarvis 1983); Winnall II (Hants) (Hawkes & Meaney 1970); Monkton Deverill (Wilts) (Rawlings 1995); Snell's Corner (Hants) (Knocker 1955); Didcot (Oxon) (Boyle et al 1995); Burghclere (Berks) (Butterworth and Loeb 1992) and SOU 862 (Southern Archaeological Services 1998) (table 1). The remaining six field cemeteries, Snell's Corner (Hants) (Knocker 1955); Ulwell (Dorset) (Cox 1989); St. Mary's Stadium (Hants) (Birbeck & Smith 2003); Bevis' Grave (Hants) (Rudkin 2001), Porchester (Hants) (Cunliffe 1976) and Cook Street (Hants) (Garner 1993;

2001; Garner & Vincent 1997), exhibited low or low-moderate levels of post-burial disturbance (table 1). Most of the post-burial disturbance observed in the field cemeteries was caused by the re-use of graves. The re-use of graves involved reopening a grave and inserting a secondary or tertiary burial, with the remains of the original occupant or occupants usually being either displaced to the sides of the grave or re-deposited above the later burial as part of the grave fill, as with the burials in graves 42 and 49 at Bevis Grave (Rudkin 2001). While the re-use of graves is generally characterised by a lack of respect towards the original occupant, occasionally care was taken not to disturb the original occupant when adding additional burials to a grave, as with burials 99 and 100 in the later churchyard at Wells Cathedral (Rodwell 2001). In this example, there is a greater level of respect towards the original occupants, and it may be that the motives that lay behind the insertion of additional burials may differ in these cases from those where the original burials are disturbed. The factors lying behind the re-use of graves is unclear. Traditionally, they have been interpreted as family plots, and in some cases, especially where later burials have been inserted with care not to disturb earlier occupants, this may be a possibility (Stoodley 2002). In many instances, however, this is unlikely due to the lack of care exhibited towards the original occupant. In these cases, the re-use either represents the accidental disturbance of earlier burials (Stoodley 2002) or purposeful re-use of earlier graves. A second form of post-burial disturbance was occasionally seen in the field cemeteries and this was caused by later burials, cutting away parts of earlier graves. This intercutting of graves usually results in part of the skeletal remains of the earlier burial being displaced while the rest remain in situ, as in grave 29 at Bevis' Grave where the upper part of the skeleton was removed by grave 28 but the lower body is undisturbed (Rudkin 2001). The bones displaced were either redeposited as part of the grave fill of the later grave or were scattered across the cemetery.

Higher levels of post-burial disturbance were observed in the majority of the churchyards, or suspected churchyards, within the study sample. Six of the eight churchyards, Barnstaple (Devon) (Miles 1984); Exeter Cathedral (Devon) (Henderson & Bidwell 1982); SOU 13 (Hants) (Morton 1992a), Staple Gardens (Hants) (Kipling & Scobie 1990); Wells Cathedral (Somset) (Rodwell 2001) and Trowbridge (Wilts) (Graham & Davies 1993) exhibited either moderate, moderate-high/high levels of post-burial disturbance. Low levels of post-burial disturbance were observed in the remaining two churchyards, Bath Abbey (Somset) (Bell 1996) and Beckery Chapel (Somset) (Rathz and Hirst 1974). There were also differences in the nature of the post-burial disturbance in the churchyard cemeteries compared with that seen in the field cemeteries. Much, and at some sites all, of the post-burial disturbances observed in field cemeteries resulted from the re-use of graves, while the

displacement of human remains due to the intercutting of graves, although present, was less common. In contrast, while there are examples of the re-use of graves from churchyards (see above), the majority of the post-burial disturbance seen in the churchyards was the result of intercutting burials. At Trowbridge, the earlier burials were interred in rows with later burials inserted between the earlier rows, a process which led to parts of the earlier burials being disturbed (Graham & Davies 1993). Similarly, the rows of burials on either side of the church at SOU 13 had been reworked five times, resulting in the redeposition of a third of all burials, with many others losing parts due to cutting by later graves (Morton 1992b). In other late cemeteries, such as Staple Gardens (Kipling & Scobie 1990), and Wells Cathedral (Rodwell 2001), the higher density of burials makes it difficult to determine the spatial layout of the cemetery and whether there was any systematic pattern to intercutting of graves.

The final major cause of post-burial disturbance of the deceased to be considered in the current study was the construction of structures associated with domestic and ecclesiastical occupation. The majority of this type of disturbance was seen in those cemeteries within the sample which lay in urban contexts, such as the middle Saxon wic site of Hamwic. The settlement contained a number of small short-lived cemeteries, the sites of which, once abandoned, were used for domestic occupation (Morton 1992b). In some cases, little time elapsed once a burial ground went out of use before the domestic occupation. For example, the earliest evidence for domestic occupation on the site of the St Mary's Stadium cemetery post-dates the graves by at most a generation (Birbeck & Smith 2003). When a cemetery was built over, the damage to the underlying burials was caused not so much by the timber domestic buildings, but by the much deeper pits associated with occupation. For example, all of the disturbed graves at St. Mary's Stadium were damaged by subsequent middle Saxon pits and not by the buildings which also overlie the site (Birbeck & Smith 2003). Usually, disturbance resulting from pits is limited to those parts of the skeleton directly cut by the pit with the rest of the skeleton remaining in situ. For example, one pit within the SOU 13 cemetery in Hamwic disturbs a grave resulting in the occupant's head being pushed back into the coffin space (Morton 1992a). The same pit also contains two isolated skulls representing disturbed remains redeposited from elsewhere (Morton 1992b). One skull is thought to belong to an adjacent grave and was probably disturbed when the pit was dug, while the origins of the other skull are unclear (Morton 1992a). Occasionally, the discovery of human remains leads to the complete excavation of the grave, as at the richly furnished St Mary's Stadium cemetery (Hants), where the discovery of one end of a grave during the middle Saxon period led to it being completely emptied, probably in the search for grave goods, with the displaced human remains being redeposited into the pit (Birbeck & Smith 2003).

The tenth and eleventh centuries saw an increasing use of stone for the construction of ecclesiastical buildings, fortifications, such as castles, and occasionally domestic buildings. These stone structures all required substantial foundation trenches, and when these buildings were associated with burial grounds, their construction could result in the substantial disturbance or destruction of human remains. The later churchyards, in particular, were prone to this type of disturbance due to the sporadic rebuilding of ecclesiastical buildings during the early medieval period, such the construction programmes associated with the tenth-century monastic reform and the Norman Conquest. The foundation trenches for the nave of Winchester's new Norman cathedral displaced approximately 1000 burials, whose remains were deposited in one of the robber trenches of the Anglo-Saxon Old Minster (Kjølbye-Biddle 1992). Similarly, the partially excavated charnel pit at Bath Abbey contained the remains of at least 33 adults, whose remains are thought to have been disturbed during the construction of the Norman abbey (Bell 1996). The Norman Conquest led not only to the rebuilding of many ecclesiastical buildings but to the appearance of castles, in both urban and rural locations. The insertion of castles into the crowded urban centres of the eleventh and early twelfth centuries was far from simple and resulted in the use of any available open space which, more often than not, was the town's burial ground. The association between late Saxon cemeteries and Norman castles is well documented (Hadley 2001) and several examples, all dating to the early twelfth century, are found in Wessex at Barnstaple (Miles 1986), Trowbridge (Graham & Davies 1993) and Taunton (Clements 1984).[1] In the case of both Trowbridge and Barnstaple, it is the defensive banks of the castle which overlie the cemetery, in effect sealing rather than disturbing the late Saxon graves (Miles 1986; Graham & Davies 1993). At Barnstaple, however, there is evidence for the reburial within a single grave of the remains of at least three bodies disturbed by the construction of the moat (Miles 1986). Whether the placing of the defensive banks may represent a conscious decision to minimise the damage to the burials caused by the construction of the castle at Barnstaple and Trowbridge is unclear. However, the fragmentary evidence from Taunton suggests that the preservation of earlier burials was not always an important consideration with the disturbed and intact remains of the occupants of the late Saxon cemetery underlying the inner and outer wards of the castle (Clements 1984).

The ultimate fate of those human remains disturbed by later activities was, by and large, governed by ease and convenience of disposal. When burials were disturbed by later graves, the displaced remains were either packed around the intrusive body or deposited into the open grave as it was backfilled. Similarly, those remains disturbed by pits or buildings were usually deposited in the nearest convenient hole in the ground, such as the pit which disturbed the burial, as at St. Mary's Stadium (Birbeck & Smith 2003), or trenches created by the robbing of stone for the new building, as at Winchester (Kjølbye-Biddle 1992). If there was nothing available, then pits may have been dug to take the displaced remains, such as at Portchester Castle where two burials thought to have been disturbed by the rebuilding of a masonry structure were reburied in small pits (Cunliffe 1976). Alternatively, in some cases, the skeletal remains were simply scattered over the site, often becoming mixed in with the rubbish (Morton 1992b). Occasionally, charnel deposits were housed in more elaborate settings, as was the case at Wells Cathedral, where a Roman mausoleum was re-used as an Anglo-Saxon ossuary (Rodwell 2001). The structure contained the remains of at least 41 individuals, and the pattern of deposition suggests that the bones were deposited over a period of time, before the structure was finally sealed in the tenth century (Rodwell 2001). The source of the bones is unclear, but the use of the ossuary as a place to deposit disturbed remains from coffins and tombs has been suggested. Finally, mention should be made of the use of disarticulated skulls as "pillow stones" in six graves at Trowbridge (Graham & Davies 1993)[2]. This behaviour mimics the later Saxon practice of placing stones around the skull (Hadley 2001).

The changing nature of post-burial disturbance in early medieval Wessex

While evidence for the post-burial disturbance of the dead in the Wessex heartlands is found throughout the early medieval period, it becomes much more prevalent in the later Saxon churchyards. However, the level of post-burial disturbance also appears to correspond to the size of the cemetery, with higher levels of disturbance tending to occur in larger cemeteries within the study sample, which are invariably associated with churches, such as Wells Cathedral (Rodwell 2001), Staple Gardens, Hants, (Kipling & Scobie 1990) and Exeter Cathedral (Henderson & Bidwell 1982). In contrast, lower levels are seen in smaller field cemeteries as well as the small late cemetery at Portchester Castle (Cunliffe 1976). Cemetery size, however, is not the only factor. While the larger of the early field cemeteries, such as Bevis Grave and Ulwell, had higher levels of disturbance than the smaller contemporary burial grounds, this was still much lower than in many of the later churchyards. The age of the site also seems to be an important factor as there are chronological differences in the nature of the post-burial disturbance. In the earlier cemeteries, the most prevalent

---

[1] Undated burials have also been found under Old Sherborne Castle (Harrison & Bayley 1977).

[2] Another two examples are found at the 4-6 Market Street site in Winchester Hampshire. The site contains part of the Cathedral cemetery, which was in use from the late tenth to early fourteenth century (Teague 1988).

type of disturbance results from the reuse of graves, with the occasional cutting of one grave by another. The pattern of disturbance seen in the later cemeteries is generally characterised by much higher levels of intercutting of graves combined with less re-use of graves, although the true level of grave re-use may, in part, be obscured by the higher levels of disturbance seen in these burial grounds. The later cemeteries, particularly those associated with churchyards, are also far more likely to have been disturbed by structural features such as buildings and pits. Finally the location of the cemetery also seems to be a factor. The majority of the cemeteries lying within urban contexts seem to be characterised by higher levels of post-burial disturbance, while the majority of rural cemeteries have much lower levels of disturbance. However, this observation needs to be qualified as the majority of rural cemeteries within this sample are small and early, while the majority of urban cemeteries are large, late and associated with churches.

The higher levels of post-burial disturbance seen in the later Saxon period are, in part, a product of the advent of churchyard burial and the impact of the increasing influence of the church over burial. However, it should also be seen, in part, as a practical response to the processes of urbanisation. The changes wrought by urbanisation are best illustrated by looking at two cemeteries from the Middle Saxon *wic* site of Hamwic. The early eighth-century cemetery at Cook Street (Hants) lies in the south-west corner of the middle Saxon settlement of Hamwic (Garner 2001). The cemetery is characterised by low levels of post-burial disturbance and well-spaced burials, although the density of burial may originally been slightly higher as there was considerable post-medieval disturbance of the site (Garner 2001). The cemetery also has many features reminiscent of the rural cemeteries of the seventh and eighth centuries (Scull 2001). The later Hamwic cemetery, SOU 13 (Morton 1992a) was in use during the eighth and ninth centuries and must have been in use only one or two generations later than the Cook Street cemetery. This cemetery has many of the features characteristic of churchyards of the medieval and post-medieval period, with a much higher density of burials, with high levels of intercut graves and post-burial disturbance (Scull 2001). The cemetery at SOU 13, unlike that at Cook Street, continued in use from after the major expansion of the settlement. This meant there was increased pressure on space within the settlement, placing the living and the dead in direct competition for space. This was a competition that the living were always going to win. The restricted space for burial meant that cemeteries, such as SOU 13, rapidly exceeded their capacity (Morton 1992b), resulting in the reworking of existing rows of burials, causing substantial post-burial disturbance in order to allow the addition of these later burials (Morton 1992b).

The increasing pressure on space within late Saxon urban centres accounts, at least in part, for the increased levels of post-burial disturbance seen in the urban cemeteries in Wessex. This fails, however, to explain the equally high levels of post-burial disturbance in the manorial cemetery at Trowbridge (Wilts) (Graham & Davies 1993). To understand the high levels, it is necessary to consider the growing influence of the Church over burial. The late Saxon period saw the increasing definition of churchyard cemeteries as fixed and separate spaces within the landscape, enclosed by boundaries and set apart by consecration (Thompson 2002). This was a custom, the documentary sources suggest that was well established by the late tenth century (Gittos 2002). The enclosing of the later churchyards is in marked contrast to the earlier field cemeteries which, in general, seem to lack boundaries with burials gradually tapering off towards their peripheries suggesting the absence of a fixed limit for burial (Gittos 2002). The enclosing of cemeteries served to restrict the space available for burial, just as efficiently as competition for space did in the urban centres, and led to the same result - high levels of post-burial disturbance as the number of burials within a cemetery exceeded its capacity. This explains the high level of post-burial disturbance at Trowbridge, as there is clear evidence for a graveyard boundary in the form of a ditch and, given the gap between the ditch and the burials, there was probably either a low bank or hedge lying just within the ditch (Graham & Davies 1993).

As has been illustrated above, the late Saxon period saw the increasing restriction of the available space for burial. This alone does not create higher levels of post-burial disturbance. Space only becomes an issue when the number of bodies exceeds the capacity of the cemetery. Even allowing for variations in the amount of the cemetery excavated, it is noticeable that the majority of the larger cemeteries listed in table 1 are of late Saxon date and these later sites are characterised by higher levels of post-burial disturbance. This raises two issues: are the chronological differences in post-burial disturbance seen in the dataset real or a function of the number of burials within a cemetery; and secondly why are the later cemeteries, in general, larger? It could be argued that the lower level of disturbance seen in the earlier cemeteries was entirely due to the small number of burials they contained. However, it should be noted that at least one early site, Bevis Grave, has more burials than the highly disturbed site of SOU 13, and, while exhibiting higher levels of disturbance than seen in many of the other earlier cemeteries, this is markedly lower than that seen at SOU 13. In addition, no evidence exists for any boundaries at Bevis Grave. Instead, the burials seem to sprawl along the ditch of the Neolithic long barrow, tapering off towards the periphery of the cemetery (Rudkin 2001). The low levels of post-burial disturbance observed at Bevis Grave suggests that higher levels of disturbance are not directly associated with the number of burials, but rather with the number of burials combined with limitations on the space available for burial. During the late Saxon period, there was a restriction of burial ground size associated with an increase in the number of burials. The latter was, in part, the result of urbanisation with the higher concentration of people found in late Saxon urban centres increasing the number of bodies. In addition, not all churches had associated cemeteries, as the right of burial was the preserve of the minster churches, albeit an increasingly contested one as the number of lay foundations mushroomed in the late tenth and eleventh centuries (Blair 1988). These restrictions on burial rights had the effect of centralising burial in rural areas at the minster church, and, in doing so, increasing the number of individuals interred within a churchyard.

Conclusion

The evidence, discussed above, demonstrates that the advent of churchyard burial in Wessex during the early medieval period ushered in high levels of post-burial disturbance of the deceased. This was due, at least in part, to the policies pursued by the Church, both by the enclosing of burial grounds and by restricting burial rights to certain churches. Initially, these policies had little effect on the levels of post-burial disturbance as churchyard burial was the preserve of ecclesiastics and those of high status. As churchyard burial become more universal, the combination of increasing numbers of bodies and a restricted amount of space available for burial resulted in escalating levels of post-burial disturbance. The Church was not the only factor, particularly in urban centres, where the pressure on space served to restrict cemetery size. The space available for burial in the earliest urban centres, such as Hamwic, was restricted due to competition long before the Anglo-Saxon Church was in a position to dictate the burial mores of the population of Wessex.

It is perhaps paradoxical that the very Church, whose policies in part caused an increase in the level of post-burial disturbance, was one with a belief in bodily resurrection (Bynum 1995). The picture painted in *Aelfric's Homilies* is one of the transformation of the physical remains of an individual on the Day of Judgement, with the surviving mortal remains playing an integral part of the process (Thompson 2002). As such, an important issue was whether the disturbance or destruction of the body after burial would prevent an individual's resurrection. According to Gregory of Tours, there was no need for concern, because on the Day of Judgement the scattered parts of bodies would be reunited (Samson 1999). In contrast, the Council of Mâcon in 585AD ruled that bodies should not be displaced to make space for later burials.[3] To some extent, the Church doctrine was rendered secondary to the practical reality which saw high levels of post-burial

disturbance in the early medieval churchyards becoming increasingly commonplace. As such, the disturbance of the dead became the accepted norm for much of the population and provided their remains lay in consecrated ground perhaps it did not matter how scattered they were.

Acknowledgments

Thanks are due to the following individuals and institutions, who have generously provided information on unpublished sites and additional information on published sites; John Allen, Barnstaple Museum, Bath Archaeological Trust, Dorset County Museum, Exeter Archaeology, Alan Morton, Portsmouth City Museum, Royal Albert Memorial Museum and Art Gallery in Exeter, David Rudkin, Graham Scobie, Somerset County Museum, Southampton City Museum, Trowbridge Museum, Wessex Trust for Archaeology, Winchester Museums Service. I would also like to thank Dawn Hadley who read and commented on various drafts of this paper. This research was funded by a University of Sheffield Studentship and the radiocarbon dating program was funded by an ORADS grant from NERC.

Literature Cited

Bell R. 1996. Bath Abbey: some new perspectives. *Bath History* 6:7-24.

Birbeck V & Smith RJC. 2003. *The origins of Middle Saxon Southampton. Excavations at St. Mary's Stadium.* 1st Draft. Unpublished manuscript held at Wessex Trust for Archaeology.

Blair J.1988. Minster churches in the landscape. In *Anglo-Saxon settlement*, Hooke, D (ed). Blackwell: Oxford; 35-58.

Boyle A, Dodd A, Miles D and Mudd A. 1995. *Two Oxfordshire Anglo-Saxon cemeteries.* Thames Valley Landscapes Monograph 8: Oxford.

Butterworth CA and Lobb SJ. 1992. *Excavations in the Burghfield area, Berkshire.* Wessex Archaeology Report No 1. Wessex Archaeology: Salisbury.

Bynum CW. 1995. *The resurrection of the body in western Christianity, 200-1336.* Columbia Press: New York.

Clements CF. 1984. The inner ward and outer bailey; burials and structures exposed in the 1970s. In *The archaeology of Taunton. Excavations and fieldwork to 1980.*, Leach, P(ed). Wessex Archaeological Trust Monograph No. 8: Salisbury; 26-32.

---

[3] Concilia Galliae A. 511-A. 695, ed C.de Clercq as referenced in Morton 1992b.

Disturbing

Corney A. 1967. A prehistoric and Anglo-Saxon burial ground, Ports Down, Portsmouth. *Proceedings of Hampshire Field Club & Archaeological Society* 24:20-58.

Cox PW. 1989. A seventh century cemetery at Shepherd's Farm, Ulwell near Swanage, Dorset. *Proceedings of the Dorset Natural History and Archaeological Society* 110:37-47.

Cunliffe BW. 1976. *Excavations at Portchester Castle. Volume II. Saxon.* Report of the Research Committee of the Society of Antiquaries of London: London.

Garner MF. 1993. Middle Saxon evidence at Cook Street, Southampton (SOU 254). *Proceedings of Hampshire Field Club & Archaeological Society* 49:77-127.

Garner MF. 2001. A middle Saxon cemetery at Cook Street, Southampton (SOU 823). *Proceedings of Hampshire Field Club & Archaeological Society* 56:170-191.

Garner MF and Vincent J. 1997. Further Middle Saxon evidence at Cook Street, Southampton (SOU 567). *Proceedings of Hampshire Field Club & Archaeological Society* 52:77-87.

Gittos H. 2002. Creating the sacred: Anglo-Saxon rites for consecrating cemeteries. In *Burial in early medieval England and Wales*, Lucy S & Reynolds A. (eds). Society for Medieval Archaeology Monograph 17. Manley Publishing: Leeds;195-208.

Graham AH and Davies SM. 1993. *Excavations in Trowbridge, Wiltshire, 1977 and 1986-1988.* Wessex Archaeology Report No. 2: Salisbury.

Hadley DM. 2001. *Death in medieval England.* Tempus: Stroud.

Harrison B and Bayley J. 1977. *Sherborne Old Castle Human Bone Report.* Ancient Monuments Laboratory Report 2451.

Henderson CG and Bidwell PT. 1982. The Saxon Minster at Exeter. In *The early church in western Britain and Ireland,* Pearce S (ed.). British Archaeological Reports (British series) 102: Oxford: BAR Publishing; 145-175.

Jarvis KS. 1983. The Bargates pagan-Saxon cemetery with late Neolithic and Bronze-Age sites. In *Excavations in Christchurch, 1969-1980*, Jarvis KS. Dorset Natural History and Archaeological Society Monograph Series, No. 5: Dorchester; 102-135

Kipling R & Scobie G. 1990. Staple Gardens 1989. Winchester Museum Service Newsletter 6:8-9.

Kjølbye-Biddle B. 1992. Dispersal or concentration: the disposal of the Winchester dead over 2000 years. In *Death in towns*, Bassett S (ed.). Leicester University Press: Leicester; 210-47.

Knocker GM.1955. Early burials and an Anglo-Saxon cemetery at Snell's Corner near Horndean, Hampshire. *Proceedings of Hampshire Field Club & Archaeological Society* 19:177-170.

Meaney A and Hawkes S. 1970. *Two Anglo-Saxon cemeteries at Winnall, Winchester, Hampshire.* Society for Medieval Archaeology Monography Series 4: London.

Miles TJ. 1984. The excavation of a Saxon cemetery and part of the Norman Castle at North Walk, Barnstaple. *Proceedings of the Devon Archaeological Society* 44:59-84.

Morton A. 1992a. *Excavations at Hamwic: Volume 1: Excavations 1946-83, excluding Six Dials and Melbourne Street.* Council for British Archaeology Research Report 84: London.

Morton A. 1992b. Burial in middle Saxon Southampton. In *Death in towns*, Bassett S (ed.). Leicester University Press: Leicester; 68-77.

Rahtz PA and Hirst SM. 1974. *Beckery Chapel Glastonbury, 1967-8.* Glastonbury Antiquarian Society: Glastonbury.

Rawlings, M. 1995. Archaeological sites along the Wiltshire section of the Codford-Ilchester water pipeline. *Wiltshire Archaeological and Natural History Magazine* 88:26-49

Rodwell, W. 2001. *Wells Cathedral. Excavations and structural studies, 1978-93.* English Heritage Archaeological Report 21: London.

Rudkin, D. 2001. *Excavations at Bevis' Grave, Camp Down, Bedhampton, Hants.* Unpublished manuscript held at Fishbourne Roman Palace Museum.

Samson, R. 1999. The church lends a hand. In *The loved body's corruption*, Downes J and Pollard T (eds.). Cruithne Press: Glasgow; 120-144.

Scull, C. 2001. Burials in emporia in England. In *Wics: The early medieval trading centres of Northern Europe*, Hill D and Cowie R (eds.). Sheffield: Sheffield University Press: Sheffield; 67-74.

Southern Archaeological Services. 1998. *Interim report on an archaeological watching brief at 75, Bitterne Road, Southampton.* Unpublished manuscript held at Southampton City Museum.

Stoodley N. 2002. Multiple burials, multiple meanings? Interpreting the early Anglo-Saxon multiple interment. In *Burial in early medieval England and Wales*., Lucy S & Reynolds A. (eds.). Society for Medieval Archaeology Monograph 17. Manley Publishing: Leeds; 103-121.

Teague SC. 1988. Excavations at Market Street 1987-88. *Winchester Museums Service Newsletter* 2:6-8

Thompson V. 2002. Constructing salvation: a homiletic and pentential context for late Anglo-Saxon burial practice. In *Burial in early medieval England and Wales*. Lucy S & Reynolds A. (eds.). Society for Medieval Archaeology Monograph 17. Manley Publishing: Leeds; 229-240.

Tallow Hill Cemetery, Worcester:
The importance of detailed study of post-mediaeval graveyards.

Alan R. Ogden,[1]* Anthea Boylston[1] and Tom Vaughan[2]

[1]Biological Anthropology Research Centre
Department of Archaeological Sciences
University of Bradford
Bradford
BD7 1DP
*e-mail address for correspondence: A.R.Ogden@bradford.ac.uk

[2]Worcestershire Historic Environment and Archaeology Service,
Woodbury,
University College Worcester
Henwick Grove
Worcester
WR2 6AJ

Abstract

Tallow Hill Cemetery, Worcester was established in an industrial part of this old cathedral city and approximately 4,800 burials took place from 1823 to 1874. A corner of this graveyard was recently excavated prior to development and two simple rectangular brick vaulted tombs were revealed along the eastern side. The first contained the burials of two children, in coffins side-by-side. The children (aged 2.0 and 3.0 years) buried in 1858 and 1863 have been identified. The second vault contained six adults, all within wooden coffins, evidently buried over a long period of time. A further burial was found in the northwest corner of the cemetery, and an unrelated human femur was retrieved from adjacent spoil.

Both children have unusually wide, round crania, with high cephalic indices, one whole standard deviation above the norm for their age, but their abnormalities do not fit an identifiable syndrome. One elderly male has perimortem saw cuts through the right side of the manubrium and the medial end of the left clavicle. These do not appear to be the result of a medical post-mortem. All 10 individuals recovered in this excavation showed obvious pathology or clear abnormalities.

It is all too frequently assumed by funding authorities that relatively recent skeletal material is of little interest, compared with more ancient bones. For this reason Victorian graveyards are often cleared commercially without careful excavation, recording and osteological investigation. However, post-mediaeval graveyards like Tallow Hill are a very rich but neglected source for the study of untreated pathology. They reveal how the present-day English population might be without late-Victorian public health measures and modern medical and dental treatment.

Keywords: Worcester, children of known age, bone saw cuts, paleopathology, congenital skull abnormalities, Victorian cemeteries.

Introduction

It has been argued that industrialization had a deleterious effect on human health, the effects of which are still being felt today (Costa 1993: Aufderheide & Rodriguez-Martin 1998). The scarcity of medieval and post-medieval cemeteries in industrial centres such as Worcester, has prevented such hypotheses from being tested.

This paper examines a post-medieval, more precisely 19th century, cemetery in Worcester. The main aim of the paper is to document the type of trauma and disease found in populations during and after the Industrial revolution.

Excavation of part of the Tallow Hill cemetery in Worcester was begun in 2002. This cemetery was established by Act of Parliament in 1792 to cope with the dramatic increase in population in Worcester in the early 19th century. This was an inner city cemetery sited in the industrial part of the city. Burials commenced in 1823 with the final interments taking place in 1895. There were approxiamately 4,700 burials, with 95 individuals interred in family vaults and brick lined graves. The initial excavation of the site identified two vaults and one deep (2.6m) burial (Vaughan 2002). In total 9 individuals and a number of disassociated bones were recovered.

The vaults contained 8 individuals, 2 children (102, 103) in one vault with 6 adults (117, 118, 127, 128, 129, 133), in the other tomb. The children were laid side by side in the N.E. corner of the first vault, one coffin directly on the floor, while the other was raised at head and foot on bricks.

The adults were all within wooden coffins. The differing styles of the coffin handles and inscription plates indicate that they were buried over a period of time, although unfortunately none of the inscription plates remained legible. It would appear that the original vaulted ceiling had collapsed at some stage after the interment of the first four individuals. The iron brackets on which two of them had been laid were buckled while the four below were sealed with a heavy layer of clay and loose bricks. This led to better preservation of the lower four (126 -129) than of the later two (117, 118) who were laid on inserted brackets above the collapse. Finally four limestone slabs had been sealed over the last interments and the tomb remortared and closed.

A further burial (126) was found in the northwest corner of the cemetery, at the unusually great depth of 2.6m. The burial had been made within a wooden coffin with iron coffin furniture. In addition a small number of unstratified bones were recovered from the adjacent spoil, including a human femur (154) and two large fragments of cattle skull.

Methods of assessment

Sex Determination

Children

The largest single problem in the analysis of immature skeletal remains is the difficulty of sexing juveniles with any degree of reliability (Schutkowski 1993; Scheuer & Black 2000). In most cases it is advisable to limit identification of sex to mature skeletons where the sources of error are significantly less (Ubelaker 1989) However, in this case the sex of the children, suggested by mandibular morphology, could be confirmed by documentation.

Adults

Sex determination, based on pelvic characteristics where possible, was carried out in adults by comparison with standards published in Bass (1987) and Buikstra and Ubelaker (1994). If the pelvis is fragmentary, other criteria can be used, but the results are less reliable. Cranial features vary between the sexes and can also be placed on a spectrum from hypermasculine to hyperfeminine. In elderly adults there is also a marked difference between the sexes in the pattern of calcification of the costal cartilages (Scheuer 1998) which can supply strong confirmatory evidence as to sex.

Age

Cranium and pelvis also provide the chief sources of information with regard to age. Pelvic methods depend on comparing degenerative changes at the joints between the pelvic bones with standards provided by casts or photographs (Iscan et al. 1984, 1985; Brooks & Suchey 1990; Lovejoy et al. 1985). With the better preserved skeletons a further aid in assessing age is the form, shape and texture of the sternal ends of the fourth ribs (Iscan et al. 1984, 1985). However, with all these ageing techniques formulae developed to give a more accurate estimation tend to overage young adults and underage the older ones (Meindl & Lovejoy 1985) and it is still quite difficult to produce an accurate estimation in the older age ranges and therefore broad categories are used when describing the age profile of an archaeological assemblage.

Stature

The estimation of living stature in archaeological populations at the present time is mainly based on the ratio of long-bone length to stature. Standards have been calculated by regression analysis based on comparison of the known living statures of American servicemen whose remains were repatriated after World War II and the Korean War, in addition to a post-mortem sample (the Terry Collection) from whom the formulae for older males and all the females have been deduced (Trotter 1970). In the present study adult stature was based whenever possible, for maximum accuracy, on the combined length of femur and tibia.

Paleopathology

Cranial and post-cranial pathological changes were recorded using macroscopic examination of bones and, where necessary, radiological examination.

Photography, Microscopy and Radiography

Calibrated photographs were taken with a Canon Coolpix 995 3.34 megapixel digital camera. Radiographs were taken in a Faxitron cabinet at 60kV using Agfa Structurix D4 film for periods of 30 – 60 seconds, depending on the density of the remaining bone.

Results

Table 1 reports the principal findings.

Identity of the individuals

None of the adults could be positively identified as their coffin plates were destroyed or illegible, and detailed cemetery records have been lost.

Table 1: The summary of the skeletal material & associated pathologies

No.	Sex	Age (years)	Site	Stature ± 3cm	Anomalies and Pathology FDI dental notation
102	male	2.0 (known)	Vault 1	NA	High cephalic index
103	female	3.0 (known)	Vault 1	NA	High cephalic index
117	male	>46	Vault 2	NA	Poor preservation Anklyosing spondylitis T4-12:L1 Osteoarthritic change L4, L5, S1 Eburnation L 1st metatarsal/proximal phalanx; R patella/distal femur Osteoporosis. Healed fracture of neck of R femur 12mm diameter hole in R temporal, probably taphonomic. Gross caries 45 and widespread cervical caries
118	female	>46	Vault 2	159cm	Spine destroyed, multiple osteolytic lesions Two lower thoracic vertebrae collapsed and wedged 4mm diameter fistula in left mastoid Gross caries of upper molars
126	male	>46	Vault 2	168cm	Only head, upper body and upper arms retrieved due to depth of burial Healed fractures to R ribs 4-8: ankylosis rib 9 Large Schmorl's nodes and osteophytes on lumbar and thoracic vertebrae Perimortem cuts to R manubrium and L clavicle Two calcified atheromatous plaques from arteries Gross caries of lower molars Upper L canine root bent through right-angle Mandibular condyles flattened, with eburnation
127	female	>46	Vault 2	165cm	Widespread osteoarthritis in hips and legs Osteoarthritis of atlanto-axial joint with eburnation of dens Osteophytes with anterior and posterior fusion of C2, C3 R jugular foramen twice the volume of L. Gross cervical caries of remaining lower anterior teeth
128	female	40-50	Vault 2	161cm	Sacralised L6 *Spina bifida occulta* S1, S2, S3 *Os acromiale* on right New bone formation on visceral surfaces of six mid-order ribs on right Gross caries 15,16,34,35,36
129	female	40-50	Vault 2	161cm	*Spina bifida occulta* S1, S2, S3 Marked asymmetry of skull base Gross caries 46
133	male	40-50	Burial	165cm	R leg & arm 7% thicker and 4% longer than left Prominent nuchal crest: large enthesophytes on limb bones Osteoarthritis of lower spine Gross caries 27,28 R mandibular condyle flattened Abrasion of L. premolars and canines from clay pipe

However the children's vault revealed a coffin plate bearing the details of a girl aged 3.0 years, who died on 7 March 1863. Burial records suggest that the other skeleton is the earlier interment of her brother, aged 2.0 years, who died on 13 March 1858. Confirmatory birth certificates, death certificates and burial records have since been found. These reveal that these individuals were the third and fourth children of a local wine merchant. The certificates record the death of the son as due to "croup" and that of the daughter as due to "measles followed by pneumonia".

Pathology and abnormalities

Congenital and developmental

Both children have unusually wide, round and bulbous crania (Figs. 1, 2), with high cephalic indices, one whole standard deviation above the norm for their ages (Farkas & Munro 1987) i.e. wider and broader than 84% of their peers. This is suggestive of some kind of congenital abnormality, but does not fit into any clearly identifiable syndrome (Olmsted 1981; Dorfman and Cerniak 1998).

In the female child there is also a smooth-walled cystic or vascular enlargement (14mm * 9mm) of the vertebral end of a 5th or 6th rib.

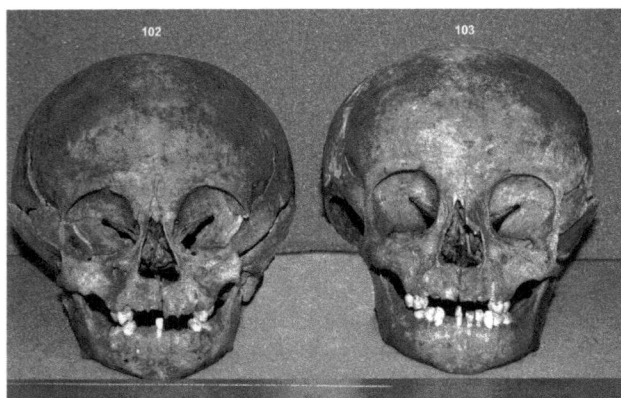

Figure 1. Anterior view of the skulls of children 102 and 103.

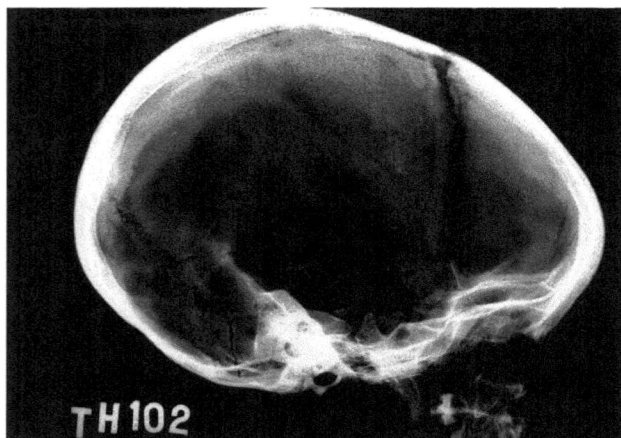

Figure 2. Lateral radiograph of skull of child 102 showing the unusually high and prominent forehead

The right jugular foramen of adult individual 127 is twice as large in area as that on the left. This is not thought to be of clinical significance (Ecinci & Unur 1997). Adult individual 129 has marked asymmetry of the skull base with unilateral asymmetrical hypoplasia of the basiocciput (Zimmerman and Kelly 1984).

Two females 128, 129, presumably related, have similarly incompletely fused sacra (*spina bifida occulta)* with involvement of sacral segments 1 to 3. The meningeal or neural structures are unlikely to have protruded through the defect, meaning that this will have been symptomless (Roberts and Manchester 1995). Individual 128 also had a sacralised sixth lumbar vertebra.

In individual 128 a separate *Os acromiale* on the right probably indicates over-rotation of the shoulder throughout childhood, preventing normal fusion with the spine of the scapula before ossification was complete.

Male 133 was clearly right-handed, as indicated by the right arm bones being 7% thicker than those on the left. But, most unusually, the right arm and leg were also 4% *longer* than those on the left. This is indicative of powerful muscular activity of those limbs in childhood and adolescence, before ossification was complete. Strenuous activity is also indicated by a strongly developed nuchal crest and prominent calcified ligamentous attachments (enthesophytes) on both olecranon prominences, superior tibiae, patellae and calcanei. There is widespread osteoarthritis of the spine, with extensive osteophytosis of the thoracic and lumbar vertebrae.

Trauma

Male 117 has gross calcification of the attachments of the *quadratus femoris* muscle, the ileo-femoral ligament and the joint capsule of the right hip secondary to a well-healed but somewhat vertically displaced fractured neck of femur. This type of fracture is sometimes traumatic, due to jumping from a height, or may be due to stress and fatigue related to running or marching (Aufderheide & Rodriguez-Martin 1998: 20). However, in this case it is probably more likely to be due to osteoporosis in old age. The bone is not sufficiently preserved for a definite diagnosis to be made.

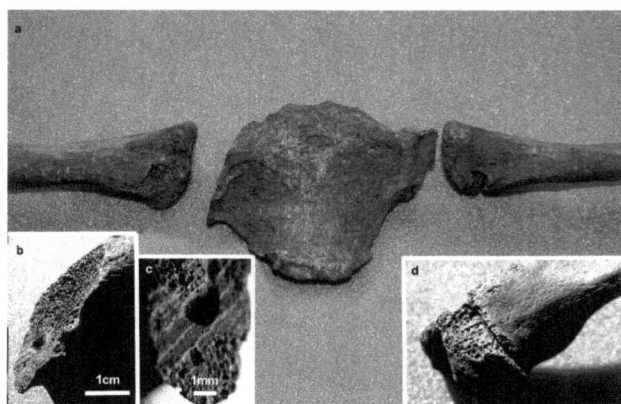

Figure 3. Manubrium and clavicles of individual 126 showing a perimortem cut to the right side of the manubrium and a partial cut to the underside of the left clavicle. Low angle lighting shows the parallel ridges produced by the sawing action of the blade.

The most puzzling aspects of individual 126 were perimortem cuts to the right side of the manubrium and the underside of the medial aspect of the left clavicle (Figure 3). Whether these were involved in his death, or were incidental to post-mortem or embalming procedures is uncertain. There are no cuts or knife marks to any of the ribs as might have been expected if a post-mortem had been performed with a reverse 'Y' incision as was usual practice at this period. (Beattie & Geiger 1987; Molleson & Cox 1993).

Photomicroscopy confirms that these are saw cuts by a fine saw-type blade, of less than 0.5mm thickness (Symes et al. 1998). If there were also cuts through the costal cartilages cannot be established, as none have survived. After discussion with other members of the osteological community, these cuts are thought most likely to be evidence of the undertakers cutting through the pectoral girdle in order to get the shoulders closer together, to wedge the body into a narrow coffin.

Individual 126 has six fractured ribs on his right side (4-9) which are all long-healed except for the last, which had failed to re-unite completely but has healed with a fibrous ankylosis.

Joint disease

Osteoarthritis

Four of the adults showed clear evidence of osteoarthritis. The most extreme example is the mature/elderly female (127) who displays severe arthritis in hips and legs. She has severe osteophytosis and anterior and posterior fusion of C2 and C3 vertebrae, with the facet joints completely fused with osteoarthritis of the atlanto-axial joint and eburnation of the *dens*. Osteophytosis is present throughout the spine.

Individuals 117 and 126 have osteophytosis of most lumbar and sacral vertebrae and 133 shows osteophytosis from T7 to L5. Male 117 also has extensive eburnation (abrasive bone-on-bone polishing) of the right patella and the distal femur, with central osteophytosis and eburnation of the left first metatarsal/proximal phalangeal joint.

Schmorl's nodes

These are the result of herniation of the intervertebral disks under heavy vertical load in early adulthood and these are seen clearly in male 126 in most thoracic and lumbar vertebrae.

Ankylosing spondylitis

Individual 117 reveals advanced *ankylosing spondylitis* (Bamboo Spine) of the lower nine thoracic and the first lumbar vertebrae (the remaining lumbar vertebrae not having survived). The fusion on the left is smooth, probably due to the presence of the aorta. On the right there are inflammatory syndesmophytes with fusion of the supraspinous ligament. Radiographs reveal the diagnostic destruction of the vertebral end-plates and the "squaring off" of the vertebral bodies. This inflammatory condition of the spine usually begins in the late teens or early twenties, starting at the sacro-iliac joints and

spreading upwards. It is commonest in European males (2.5:1 male:female) and in modern populations can occur in up to 1% of the population. It is produced by inflammatory changes in the bony insertions of the *annulus fibrosus*, the outer fibrous ring of the intervertebral disks. The clinical features of this condition are stiffness, lower back pain, fatigue and weight loss. Severe limitation of chest movement leads to sharp pleuritic chest pain, fibrosis of the lungs, a trebling of the risk of respiratory disease and a predisposition to heart disease (Calin 1993). Other arthritic change, to be expected in 20-40% of sufferers is revealed by severe osteoarthritis of the right knee and left foot in this individual. The porotic nature of most of the bones of this male, with almost complete loss of cancellous bone may be taphonomic, but is also probably partly due to osteoporosis secondary to the *ankylosing spondylitis* (Will et al. 1989).

Infectious disease

Non-specific infection

Dental abscesses were common, with gross dental caries and pulpal exposure in at least one tooth in every adult (described in more detail in the section on dental pathology).

A large 4mm diameter fistula in the left mastoid of individual 118 indicates long-term chronic infection and pus drainage from her mastoid sinus.

Specific infections

Tuberculosis

A large and very clear area of periosteal new bone formation on the visceral surfaces of six middle order right ribs in female 128 indicates severe prolonged lung infection and pleurisy. In recent years, lesions of the ribs have attracted increasing attention from paleopathologists as potential indicators of tuberculosis, but recent work with DNA has questioned this (Mays et al. 2002). The authors state that visceral surface rib lesions should simply be considered nonspecific indicators of intrathoracic infection, unless linked with evidence from other bones. There are no other specific features in this skeleton suggestive of tuberculosis, but public health records show that pulmonary tuberculosis, otherwise known as "consumption" or "phthisis" was the commonest cause of death by single disease in the early Nineteenth Century (Aufderheide & Rodriguez-Martin 1998: 130).

Unstratified bone found in the spoil heap includes a solitary human adult left femur (154) with its head destroyed by arthritic or tuberculous change and with an atrophied proximal shaft which indicates long-term loss of function as a load-bearing limb.

Metabolic and endocrine disorders

Osteoporosis

This was seen in two individuals; male 117, secondary to *ankylosing spondylitis*, and female 118, at least partially the result of widespread metastases.

Neoplastic disease

Individual 118 is the poorly preserved adult skeleton of a female, aged at least 50 with most vertebral bodies missing, and with multiple rounded osteolytic lesions, probably neoplastic metastases, in the remaining vertebral spinous and transverse processes (Zimmerman & Kelly 1984). Radiographs support this diagnosis. However radiological features of skeletal metastases are generally not diagnostic as to the site of the primary tumour. The commonest primary sites for osteolytic lesions in women are breast, uterus and ovary (Greenspan & Remagen 1998). The appearance and distribution of the lesions in this particular skeleton is very similar to that reported by Mays et al. (1996) and Sefcatova et al. (2001). There is general osteoporosis, and therefore little arthritic change, but two lower thoracic vertebrae have partially collapsed and are wedged, though whether because of osteoporosis or metastases is difficult to be sure.

Osteolytic metastases of carcinoma are nowadays by far the most common skeletal manifestation of malignant disease (Dorfman & Czerniak 1998). However only 76 similar cases have been described in the whole of old-world archaeology (Sefcatova et al. 2001), revealing how rare this condition is in archaeological populations. Malignant disease would be expected to be much more common in post-medieval populations, though whether this is because of more people living to greater ages, or increased levels of carcinogens in the environment, is a matter of debate (Aufderheide & Rodriguez-Martin 1998).

Dental disease

There is gross dental caries with pulpal exposure in at least one tooth in each adult and heavy calculus deposits are common amongst the older individuals. The levels of caries in most individuals from Tallow Hill are high. Although the prevalence is higher in the molar teeth (47%), levels of caries are high even in the more anterior teeth (18%). The severity of the caries in half of all remaining molars and the lack of severe periodontal disease suggests that most extractions had been because of caries. This indicates that the true overall incidence of caries is 45%, and that individuals were living on a highly cariogenic diet. It is interesting that the minimal amount of dental wear seen in these individuals is similar to modern levels. In other words, their diet was relatively unabrasive, fine-ground and sticky compared with diets in earlier periods. For this reason ageing these individuals

by their tooth wear (Brothwell 1981) suggested ages some ten to fifteen years younger than did the other skeletal age indicators. The general poor state of dental health from this time period is widely known (Whittaker 1993).

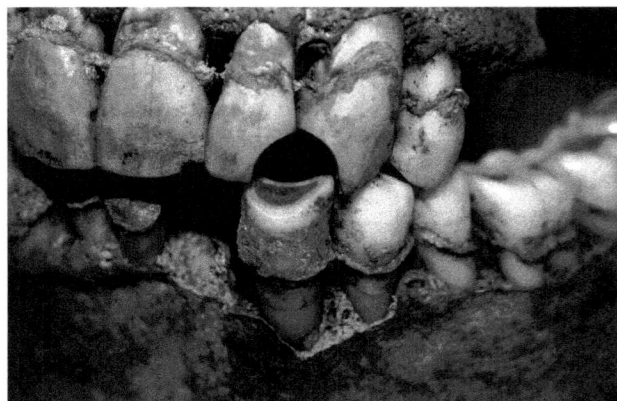

Figure 4. Individual 133 shows the classical smooth wear produced by the round stem of a clay pipe. The formation of secondary dentine has prevented exposure and infection of the dental pulps of the three teeth involved.

One male (133) was a clay pipe smoker, revealed by the characteristic polished oval voids worn between his opposing lateral incisor and canine teeth, on both sides (Figure 4). His right mandibular condyle is flattened, compared with that on the left and this may be due to asymmetrical occlusal loading. By contrast in individual 126 both mandibular condyles are flattened with small areas of eburnation. This is probably due to overclosure of the mandible by the powerful jaw muscles once the mobile teeth could no longer produce a solid occlusal contact.

Discussion

There are many problems involved in the analysis of disease from dry bone. The first is that many of the pathological conditions that can affect individuals and have a significant impact on their daily lives, possibly even leading to death, leave no traces on the skeleton. Acute infectious conditions, which in an era before the advent of antibiotics would have been more likely to lead to the death of individuals, tend not to leave skeletal markers. The diseases that affect the skeleton are more likely to be chronic conditions of long-standing. Where changes do occur on bones, the problem is that there are only a limited number of ways in which bone can react to pathogens (new bone formation, resorption, or a combination of the two) and as such, it can be difficult to diagnose conditions observed. When skeletons are poorly preserved, as two were in this case, it can make the task of determining the cause of changes very difficult. Pathological changes reported in skeletal material should therefore be taken as a minimum of the amount of pathology and trauma that may have affected the individuals during life, and uncertainty over differential diagnoses is inevitable.

The death of the female child from the complications of measles is a salutary reminder, in view of the present day controversy over the low take-up of the Measles, Mumps and Rubella (MMR) vaccination, that children can be seriously damaged or even die of measles and its complications.

It is significant that every single individual retrieved from Tallow Hill Cemetery showed obvious pathology or clear abnormalities. This was in spite of the fact that eight of the individuals came from private vaults and so were presumably from wealthy and well-connected families. This study has illustrated that post-Medieval graveyards may be a rich and valuable source for the study of untreated pathology.

It is all too often assumed by funding authorities that relatively recent skeletal material is of little interest, compared with more ancient bones. For this reason Victorian graveyards are often cleared commercially without careful excavation, recording and osteological investigation. It is salutary to consider that these cemeteries perhaps reveal how the present-day English population would be without late Victorian public health measures, fluoride toothpastes and modern medical and dental treatment. The scarcity of detailed studies of Victorian graveyards such as Tallow Hill prevents direct assessment of the impact of industrialisation on human health. This is of great importance, as the long-term effects of the urban and industrial revolutions are still being worked out in modern-day society.

Conclusions

All 10 individuals retrieved from Tallow Hill Burial Ground showed obvious pathology or clear abnormalities. This excavation illustrates that post-Mediaeval graveyards are a rich source for the study of untreated pathology and perhaps reveal how the present-day population of Worcester would be without late Victorian public health measures and modern medical and dental treatment.

Acknowledgements

The authors are very grateful to Dr Christopher Knüsel and Dr Darlene Weston of the University of Bradford for the considerable help and encouragement they have given to this project; and to Helen Curtis who supplied the much of the information on the history of Tallow Hill Cemetery.

Literature Cited

Aufderheide AC and Rodriguez-Martin C (1998) *The Cambridge Encyclopedia of Human Paleopathology.* Cambridge: Cambridge University Press.

Barnes E (1994) *Developmental defects of the axial skeleton in Paleopathology*. Colorado: University Press.

Bass WM (1987) *Human osteology: a laboratory and field manual.* Missouri: Missouri Archaeological Society.

Beattie O and Geiger J (1987) *Frozen in Time: The fate of the Franklin Expedition.* London: Bloomsbury Publishing.

Brooks S and Suchey JM (1990) Skeletal age determination based on the os pubis: a comparison of the Acsádi-Nemeskéri and Suchey-Brooks methods. *Human Evolution* 5: 227-238.

Brothwell DR. (1965) *Digging up bones*. Ithaca, New York: Cornell University Press

Buikstra JE and Ubelaker DH (1994) *Standards for data collection from human skeletal remains.* Fayetteville: Arkansas Archeological Survey Research Series 44.

Calin A (1993) Ankylosing spondylitis. In PJ Maddison, DA Isenberg, P Woo, and DN Glass (eds.): *Oxford Textbook of Rheumatology.* Oxford: Oxford University Press.

Costa DL (1993) Height, weight and disease among native-born in the rural antebellum North. *Social Science History* 17: 355-383.

Dorfman H and Czerniak B (1998) *Bone Tumours.* St Louis: Mosby.

Ecinci N and Unur E (1997) Macroscopic and morphometric investigation of the jugular foramen of the human skull. *Anatomical Science International* 72: 525-529.

Farkas LG and Munro IR (1987) *Anthropomorphic proportion in Medicine.* Springfield: Charles C. Thomas.

Greenspan A. and Remagen W (1998) *Differential diagnosis of tumors and tumor-like lesions in bones and joints.* Philadelphia: Lippincott-Raven.

Isçan MY, Loth SR, Wright RK. (1984) Age estimation from the rib by phase analysis: white males. *Journal of Forensic Science* 29: 1094-1104.

Isçan MY, Loth SR, and Wright RK (1985) Age estimation from the rib by phase analysis: white females. *Journal of Forensic Science* 30: 853-863.

Lovejoy CO, Meindl S, Przybeck TR, and Mensforth BP (1985) Chronological metamorphosis of the auricular surface of the ilium. A new method for the determination of skeletal age at death. *American Journal of Physical Anthropology* 68: 15-28.

Mays S, Fysh E, Taylor GM (2002) Investigations of the link between visceral surface rib lesions and tuberculosis in a medieval skeletal series from England using ancient DNA. *American Journal of Physical Anthropology* 119: 27-36.

Mays S, Strouhal E, Vyhnanek L, and Nemeckova A (1996) A case of metastatic carcinoma of medieval date from Wharram Percy England. *Journal of Paleopathology* 8: 33-42.

Meindl R and Lovejoy C (1985) Ectocranial suture closure: A revised method for the determination of skeletal age at death. *American Journal of Physical Anthropology* 68: 57-66.

Molleson T and Cox M (1993) *The Spitalfields project: Volume 2: The anthropology: The middling sort.* CBA Research Report 86: York: Council for British Archaeology.

Olmsted WM (1981) *Some skeletogenic lesions with common calvarial manifestations.* Radiologic Clinics of North America 19: 703.

Roberts C and Manchester K (1995) *The archaeology of disease.* Ithaca, New York: Cornell University Press; 36.

Scheuer L (1998) Age at death and cause of death of the people buried in St Bride's Church, Fleet Street London. In M Cox (ed.): *Grave concerns: death and burial in England 1700-1850.* CBA Research Report 113, York: Council for British Archaeology: 100-111.

Scheuer L and Black S (2000) *Developmental juvenile osteology.* San Diego: Academic Press.

Schutkowski H (1993) Sex determination of infant and juvenile skeletons: 1. Morphognostic features. American *Journal of Physical Anthropology* 90: 199-205.

Sefcatova A, Strouhal E, and Nemeckova A (2001) Case of metastatic carcinoma from end of the 8th – early 9th Century Slovakia. *American Journal of Physical Anthropology* 116: 216-229.

Symes SA, Berryman HE, and Smith O (1998) Saw marks in bone: introduction and examination of residual kerf contour. In Reichs K. (ed.). *Forensic Osteology: Advances in the identification of human remains.* Charles C. Thomas: Springfield, Illinois. 389-409.

Trotter M (1970) Estimation of stature from intact long bones. In TD Stewart (ed.): *Personal identification in mass disasters.* Washington DC: Smithsonian Institution Press; 71-83.

Ubelaker DH. (1989) *Human skeletal remains: excavation analysis interpretation.* 2nd edn. Washington: Taraxacum; 52.

Vaughan T (2002) *Archaeological watching brief at Tallow Hill, St. Martins, Worcester.* Archaeological Service, Worcester: Worcester County Council.

Whittaker D (1993) Oral Health. In T Molleson and M Cox (eds.): *The Spitalfields Project: The Anthropology: the middling sort.* York: Council for British Archaeology Research Report 86; 49-65.

Will R, Palmer R, Bhalla AK, Ring F, and Calin A (1989) Marked osteoporosis is present in early ankylosing spondylitis and may be a primary pathological event. *Lancet* ii; 1483-1484.

Zimmerman MR. and Kelly MA (1984) *Atlas of human paleopathology.* New York: Praeger; 126-127.

Heads, Shoulders, Knees and Toes
Human Skeletal Remains from Raven Scar Cave in the Yorkshire Dales

Stephany Leach

Department of Archaeology, University College Winchester
Sparkford Road
Winchester
SO22 4NR
Stephany.leach@winchester.ac.uk

Abstract

Human skeletal remains from Raven Scar Cave were reanalysed in order to determine the function of the site and the agents involved in site formation processes. Only minimal direct anthropological analysis has been carried out on this material in recent years. Assumptions and ideas were formulated decades ago with little regard to the human remains. This cave site was thought to represent a burial area for more than twenty Later Neolithic individuals, originally interred in simple slab-and-boulder built cists.

Reanalysis of the osteological material from this site suggested a minimum number of fifteen individuals. The death assemblage predominantly consisted of children and young adults. Skeletal part representation and bone surface modifications were not indicative of whole body inhumations, suggesting that the function of this cave site was not simply a repository for burial. Animal scavenging from exposed corpses in the vicinity and human manipulation of body parts, particularly the crania, seems a more likely interpretation of the excavated human remains.

Keywords: Cave, Later Neolithic, Animal Scavenging, Fragmentation, Head Cult, Mummification.

Introduction

There has been considerable interest in caves and cave archaeology during the last two centuries. In the 19th century caves were recognised as unique repositories of archaeological and palaeoenvironmental evidence (Dawkins 1874; Smith 1865). During the 1930s to 1970s further interest in cave sites in Yorkshire resulted in a series of excavations in the region, although few publications (Gilks 1989, 1988; Fitton & Mitchell 1950; Simpson 1950). However, after this period the focus of interest shifted and British caves became marginalised as a subject of serious study.

Caves are fascinating features within the landscape. Folklore narratives and ethnographic studies highlight the importance of cave use and perception by various cultures (Bonsall & Tolan-Smith 1997; Bradley 2000). Neglect of the archaeological record derived from these sites has resulted in a lack of recognition of the key and unique role caves played in landscape development and interaction.

The co-occurrence of Neolithic monumental burial and cave burial practices has led to the suggestion that cave burial represented a lower status or an ordinary form of burial, while the monuments were reserved for the privileged few (Chamberlain 1997). Among the death assemblages excavated from these locations, a larger proportion of subadult remains were recovered from the cave sites than the monuments. This assumption, that caves represented a lower status burial arena, may have contributed to their marginalisation as a focus of archaeological interest.

An alternative explanation for burial in caves has been proposed by King (2001). He suggests the dispersed nature of the skeletal remains across the landscape, in natural locations such as caves, should be viewed as the consequence of mobile occupation and random incidents of 'death and discard' across the landscape. These assemblages need not be seen as the result of a specific elaborate or intentional ritual but rather the 'fallout' relating to subsistence and residential habits. According to this theory, cave burial is a straightforward solution to a problem of disposal.

Most of the human skeletal material from caves in the Yorkshire region is considered to be prehistoric, either Neolithic or Bronze Age, and derived from articulated burials (Gilks 1989). Initial research for the current study was based on the assumption that these individuals represented the strata of society that were not included in the prestigious burial monuments. The assemblage was re-analysed with a view to understanding the reasons for their exclusion from more formal burial contexts.

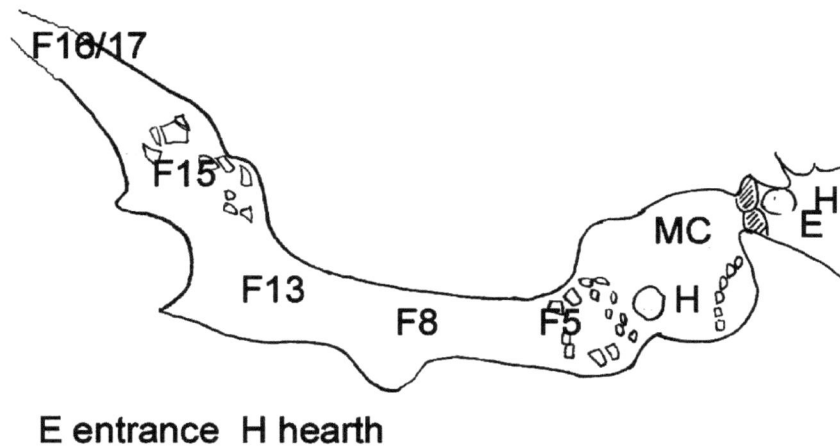

Figure 1: Sketch Plan of Raven Scar Cave

Raven Scar Cave

Raven Scar Cave is located in the Yorkshire Dales. The small, concealed entrance to the cave is located high up in the steep face of the scar. From the entrance or main chamber, a narrow passage runs almost horizontally to the back of the cave (Figure 1). Following discovery in 1973, nine short seasons resulted in the complete excavation of the cave (Gilks 1976). The location and context of finds were recorded in detail and it has been possible to reconstruct the site with regard to the spatial layout of the skeletal material and thereby gain an understanding of the site formation processes. Finds from Raven Scar include a Middle or Early Bronze Age bronze disc-headed pin, a bone whistle, flint scrapers, a plano-convex knife, a tanged and barbed arrowhead, an amber bead and a spindle whorl. The pottery includes Late Neolithic, All-Over-Cord Beaker (AOC) and part of an Early Bronze Age Collared Urn (Gilks 1976, 1985). Gilks considered that the human remains clearly attest to the site being used as a cemetery with two phases of burial activity indicated (Gilks 1976: 98) involving more than twenty burials, all of which had originally been interred in slab-and-boulder built cists (Gilks 1989: 12).

Methodology

Each assemblage of bones is, to a certain degree, taphonomically and biologically unique. The aim of this study was to use a combined methodology, utilising both taphonomic and anthropological data to reanalyse this collection. Through this approach it may be possible not only to reconstruct circumstances relating to the site formation processes and the agents involved, but also to consider some of the reasons for selection or deposition of the individuals represented in this assemblage.

The skeletal material from this cave site was disarticulated, commingled and quite fragmented. To record as much detail as possible, an individual specimen recording system was used. Each bone or bone fragment was given a specimen number and the taphonomic characteristics were recorded. If the fragment was identifiable to a particular element, a supplementary form was completed to document the biological characteristics. These recording sheets formed the basis of the osteological profile for the site. The material was laid out in order or sequence of cave topography and refitting of specimens was attempted. This provided valuable information with regard to the movement of elements and fragments within the cave.

Six stages of bone weathering, as defined by Behrensmeyer (1978), were employed to classify the level of exposure exhibited by each fragment. Surface abrasion or smoothing was also noted. The fragments were examined for evidence of animal chewing and human processing, such as cut marks. The number and characteristics of bone fractures were recorded. These included the location, type or outline and the surface contour of the fracture. The colour and texture of the fracture surface and the presence of internal bevelling in cranial fractures were also noted. Examples used as a reference for this analysis include those illustrated by Larsen (1997: 135), Lovell (1997: 142-143) and Villa and Mahieu (1991: 35-36). Antemortem fractures were not included in this section, but suspected perimortem trauma was recorded. The morphology of the fracture, the outline and angle, may provide an indication of the timing of the fracture event and the type of force involved.

Table 1: Raven Scar Cave skeletal element representation by minimum number of elements (MNE)

	Main Chamber (MC & F4)	Passage, front (F5, F8 & F13)	Passage, mid (F15)	Passage, rear (F16 & F17)	Total MNE
Loose teeth	86	5	6	6	103
Cranium/Maxilla	1	2	1	-	4
Mandible	2	3	1	2	8
Cervical vertebra	-	-	1	1	2
Thoracic vertebra	2	4	-	-	6
Lumbar vertebra	-	-	-	-	-
Sacrum	-	-	-	-	-
Pelvis	-	-	-	-	-
Sternum	-	-	-	-	-
Rib	4	17	7	12	40
Clavicle	3	-	1	1	5
Scapula	1	1	1	1	4
Humerus	-	-	1	3	4
Radius	-	3	-	1	4
Ulna	-	2	1	4	7
Carpal	-	-	-	-	-
Metacarpal	-	2	1	4	7
Phalanx (hand)	9	1	-	8	18
Femur	2	-	-	-	2
Patella	-	-	-	1	1
Tibia	3	1	-	1	5
Fibula	3	2	-	4	9
Tarsal	-	-	-	2	2
Metatarsal	-	-	-	6	6
Phalanx (foot)	-	-	1	2	3

The extent and intensity of fracturing in the assemblage was calculated by relating the number of fragments or specimens (NISP) to the minimum number of elements (MNE) identified, the NISP being higher in fragmented remains. As fragmentation serves to reduce the capacity of a specimen to be identified, analytical absence of skeletal parts may result from high intensity fracturing and is equivalent to the actual destruction of a skeletal element even though fragments remain (Lyman 1994: 379). Intensive fragmentation will ultimately reduce the minimum number of elements and, therefore, individuals within the assemblage. Accordingly, when element representation within the cave was compared, the level of fragmentation was considered. The minimum number of each skeletal element was calculated for the assemblage and for zones or areas within the site. Skeletal element representation and frequency constitutes the basic analytical structure or character of this assemblage.

Categories of biological data recorded include: age at death estimation; sex assignment; metric and non-metric traits; musculoskeletal stress markers and other activity indicators; growth, developmental and nutritional stress indicators, trauma and pathologies. Although the cave skeletal assemblage was disarticulated and commingled, the basic principles of age at death estimations and sex assignment were applied to the relevant elements (Bass 1987; Buikstra & Ubelaker 1994; Chamberlain 1994). Dental wear stages were recorded (Smith 1984). Age at

death for the subadult material in this assemblage was estimated using dental development and eruption stages (Moorees et al. 1963a, 1963b; Smith 1991), the appearance of centres of ossification and fusion (Krogman & Iscan 1986; McKern & Stewart 1957; Suchey et al. 1984) and diaphyseal length (Hoffman 1979; Scheuer et al. 1980; Ubelaker 1989). The cranial and postcranial skeletal elements were subjected to the standard series of measurements (Bass 1987; Brothwell 1981).

Results

Due to the level of finds recording and contextual information, it has been possible to construct individual osteological profiles for specific areas within the cave. Much of the skeletal material exhibited evidence of carnivore chewing (Figures 2 and 3) and certain regions of the body were not represented in the assemblage. As the cave had been completely excavated and small elements were present, including those susceptible to differential preservation, their absence would appear to be a genuine characteristic of this assemblage. A total of 424 identified specimens (NISP) were recorded, the minimum number of elements (MNE) was 240. From the postcranial material, a minimum number of four individuals was calculated. With the exception of two lower cervical vertebrae and six subadult vertebral arches, the spinal column, sacrum, pelvic bones and sternum

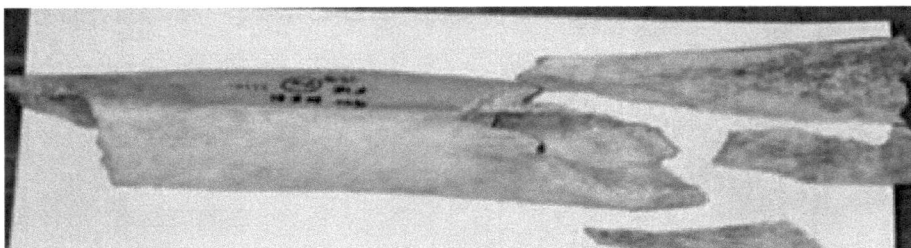

Figure 2: Tibia exhibiting evidence of carnivore chewing

were not represented, even in fragmentary form. Apart from some fragmentary ribs, the thoracic and pelvic region of the body appeared absent. Although the MNE provided a minimum estimate of four individuals, the dental evidence indicated a higher estimate of individuals represented. A significant number of loose teeth were excavated from the main chamber, which, combined with the *in situ* teeth of eight mandibles and two maxillae, provided a minimum number estimate of fifteen individuals.

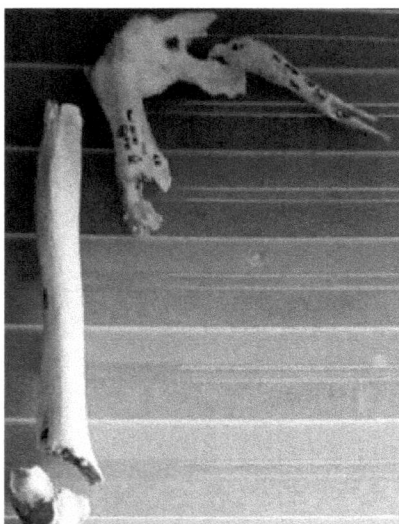

Figure 3: Evidence of carnivore chewing from area F15

Individual skeletal profiles were constructed for specific areas within the cave. The assemblage was subdivided into the following six zones: Main Chamber; F5; F8; F13; F15 and F16/17. These areas are marked on the sketch plan of the cave's features in Figure 1 and represent sections of the cave running from the entrance to the innermost part of the cave. Taphonomic and biological characteristics of the skeletal sub-assemblages varied markedly. The MNE for the cave assemblage and sub-assemblages are presented in Table 1. The most predominant characteristic of this assemblage is the large quantity of loose teeth in the Main Chamber.

Bone fracture characteristics of the assemblage are presented in Tables 2 and 3. A higher proportion of characteristics that imply the bone was fresh when broken occur in the far passage of the cave. Variation in bone surface modifications, in relation to specific zones, was also noted (Table 4). There was little evidence for animal modifications in the main chamber. Evidence of carnivore activity was focused towards the back of the cave in the passage leading from the main chamber. Targets for carnivore attention included the long bones of the upper extremities, the tibia and fibula, the clavicle and scapula, metatarsals and ribs. Specimens, from these contexts, that displayed no evidence of carnivore or rodent activity consisted mostly of bones of the hand, ankle and foot.

Table 2: Raven Scar Cave outline characteristics of long bone fractures(percentage NISP)

	Main Chamber (MC&F4)	Passage front (F5,8&13)	Passage Mid F15	Passage rear (F16&17)
Transverse / Curved	53	43	17	29
Spiral / V	41	36	50	50
Jagged	6	21	33	16
Longitudinal	-	-	-	5
Total	100	100	100	100

The bone weathering pattern exhibited by specimens in the various contexts demonstrated a distinct division between bones in the main chamber and those in the rear passage. Elements in the main chamber exhibited weathering stage 1 or 2, those deposited in the passage all exhibited weathering stage 0. It would appear that the bones towards to the back of the cave were not exposed to the elements. Those in the main chamber experienced some degree of exposure, perhaps due to its proximity to the entrance and the lack of immediate burial of these elements.

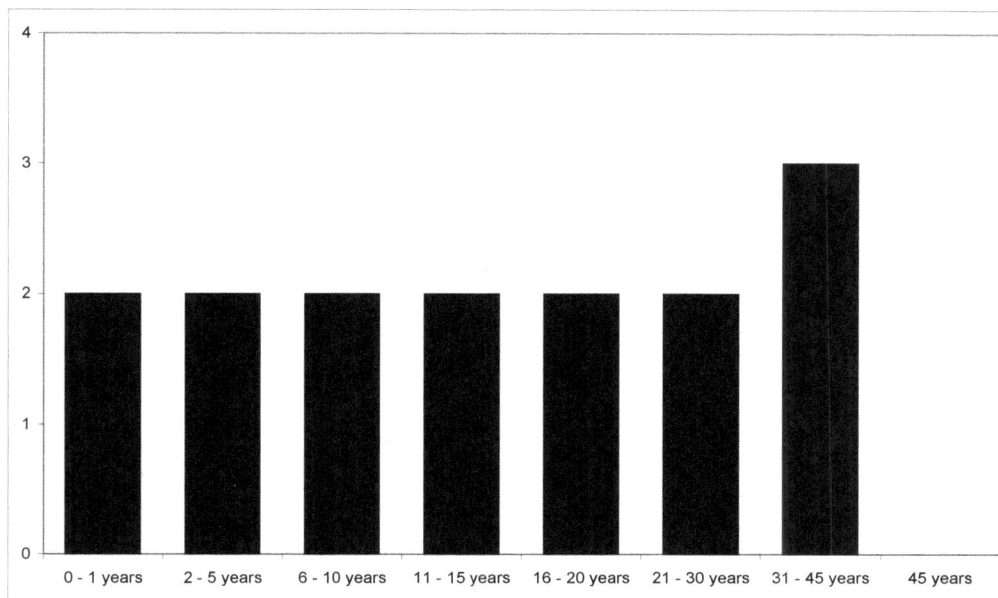

Figure 4: Raven Scar Cave age at death profile

Table 3: Raven Scar Cave surface characteristics of long bone fractures (percentage NISP)

	Main Chamber	Pass. front	Pass. mid	Pass. rear
Oblique	44	54	50	73
Right-angle	56	46	50	27
Total	100	100	100	100

Approximately 85% of the loose dentition excavated from Raven Scar Cave derived from the main chamber. According to the original excavation plan, they appear to have been randomly dispersed. The combined tooth count including *in situ* permanent and deciduous dentition from eight mandibles and two maxillae totalled 199 (of which 134 were mandibular and 65 maxillary). Of the loose teeth, 63% were mandibular, 37% maxillary. Calculations to estimate the minimum number of individuals (MNI) at this site were based on the number of teeth classified according to tooth type, side and developmental stage. The MNI represented by the dentition was fifteen, based on eleven mandibular left 1st premolars and 4 children who died before premolar development was complete.

As the vast majority of human remains represented in this assemblage were teeth, age estimates were mainly established using tooth development, eruption stages and attrition. Due to the destruction of diaphyseal ends and loss of epiphyses through carnivore activities, the age structure of the subadult death assemblage is based primarily on the dentition. Estimation of age at death and sex assignment for the adults represented in the Raven Scar assemblage was problematic. Degenerative changes in the pelvic bones provide the primary indicators of age at death, but these elements were entirely absent from this collection. Similar difficulties were experienced in the assignment of sex due to the lack of these elements. Damage to the ends of long bones, caused by carnivores, removed metric evidence relating to joint dimensions used to supplement secondary sexual morphological characteristics. The crania and mandibles formed the only source of evidence available, but these were often fragmentary. Of the five individuals aged over twenty years at death, two were possibly female and two possibly male. The age profile of the assemblage is illustrated in Figure 4.

Table 4: Raven Scar Cave bone surface modification agents NISP (%)

	Main chamber	Pass. front	Pass. mid	Pass. rear
None	112 (95)	97 (94)	15 (39)	97 (59)
Human	2 (2)	-	1 (3)	-
Carnivore	4 (3)	2 (2)	21 (55)	63 (38)
Rodent	-	-	-	-
Carnivore & Rodent	-	4 (4)	1 (3)	5 (3)
Total	118 (100)	103 (100)	38 (100)	165 (100)

Discussion

Gilks (1976: 96) has stated that the human remains excavated from Raven Scar Cave clearly attest to the site being exploited for burials and then sealed to exclude predators. He further stated (1989:12) that the cave produced the remains of more than twenty Later Neolithic burials, all of whom had originally been interred in simple, unroofed, slab-and-boulder built cists. Following a careful and detailed analysis of the skeletal material, a minimum number estimate of fifteen individuals was calculated for the site. Furthermore, the nature of the skeletal assemblage indicates that the practice of whole body burials at this site was unlikely. Gilks also suggested that, after a certain level of decomposition, some of the skeletal elements were removed to make way for later interments or to use the area for a different purpose (1976: 98). This activity may have occurred, although traces of the absent elements of the spinal column and pelvic girdle should be represented in the assemblage. Human manipulation of body parts usually involves the crania or long bones rather than this section of the body. The selective, secondary deposition of skeletal elements in the cave may have produced these anomalies in skeletal representation. However, the presence of small bones, such as phalanges of the hands and feet, usually do not form the focus of this type of selective deposition. Differential preservation of this area of the body also seems unlikely due to the presence of these smaller more fragile elements.

The presence of carnivore modification, on the surface of the bones in the passage beyond the main chamber, may provide a clue to at least one of the agents involved in the site formation process. Once the characteristics of the skeletal representation of this assemblage were established, it was suggested that carnivores may have entered the cave and disturbed the burials within (T Lord pers. comm.). However, carnivore disturbance of cave burials did not account for the missing elements or regions of the body.

Haglund (1997a) has identified the characteristic stages and sequence of disarticulation of the human corpse by carnivores. He has identified the elements or sections of the body that often become detached from the corpse and carried away by the animal for consumption. This pattern of skeletal dismemberment and dispersal occurred when the body was left exposed on the ground surface; shallow burial, bodies heavily clothed or placed inside a structure modified this pattern (Haglund et al. 1989:594).

The removal pattern of bones or articulated groups of bones during carnivore scavenging is illustrated in Figure 5. There are some striking similarities when compared with the skeletal elements excavated from the cave. This, together with the presence of carnivore modification on the bones in the cave passage, strongly suggests the agency of carnivores in the site formation process. It

would seem likely that scavenging animals were dismembering and dispersing body parts from corpses left exposed in the vicinity. It does not, however, preclude other activities or agents, as there are certain anomalies to this pattern in the assemblage.

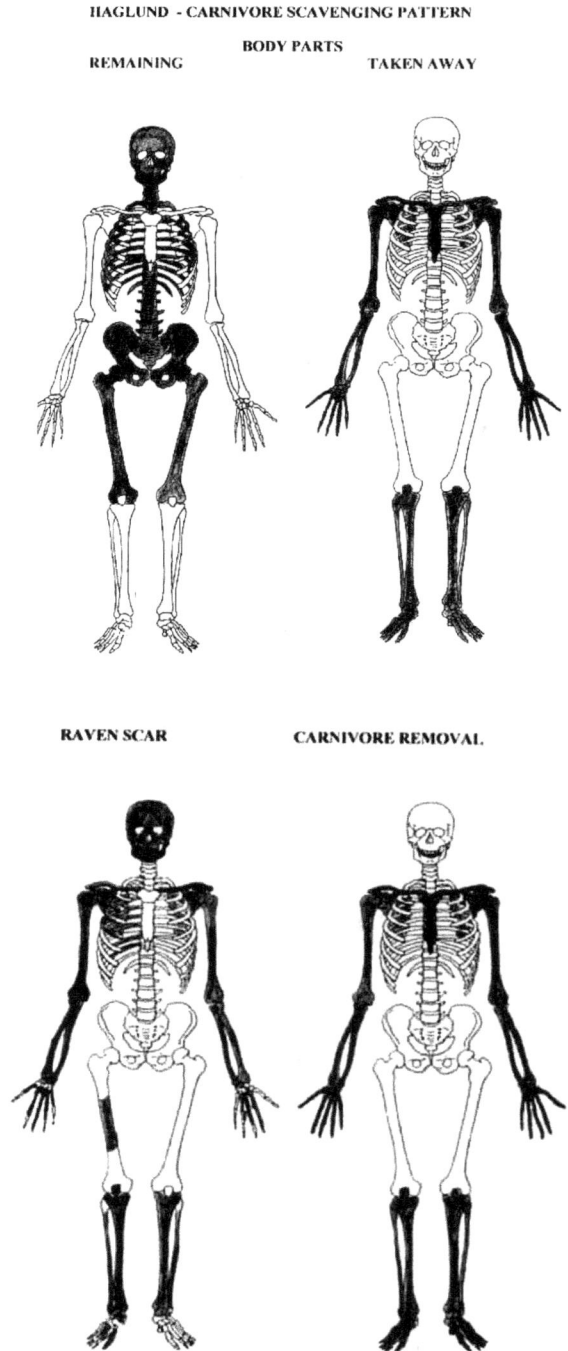

Figure 5: Comparison of carnivore scavenging behaviour with the assemblage from Raven Scar Cave (adapted from Haglund 1997a:376

By identifying non-human site formation processes, human action or manipulation of body parts or skeletal elements may be highlighted. The most striking anomaly, or deviation from the animal scavenging skeletal pattern, is the presence of the crania, eight mandibles and a substantial amount of loose dentition scattered in the main chamber. These elements are not usually transported away by animals from the original site of deposition. Calculation of the minimum number of individuals indicated a disparity between the different elements: a MNI of 4 was calculated for the crania, 8 for the mandible and 15 for the teeth. Two thirds of these individuals represented appear to be under the age of 20.

A proportional excess of anterior teeth in the loose teeth assemblage was highlighted. Single-rooted teeth separate from their sockets early in the decomposition process (Haglund 1997b: 383). As decomposition progresses, the mandible then becomes detached from the cranium. The human skeletal and dental evidence from Raven Scar may indicate that a minimum of fifteen, possibly isolated, heads were taken into the cave's main chamber. These seem to have been left for a certain period of time while decomposition progressed to varying degrees, resulting in the loss of mostly single-rooted anterior teeth. The mandibles of some of the crania also became detached, remained in the cave and became dispersed, possibly by a second agent. The presence and frequency of human elements in this assemblage suggests that fleshed skulls were brought into the main chamber of this cave. The entrance may have been blocked to protect them, but after a period of time, during which a level of decomposition resulted in the separation or loss of certain elements, the crania were then removed. The lack of upper cervical vertebrae in the cave assemblage would indicate that some soft tissue remained when the crania were removed – in the disarticulation sequence, the mandible detaches prior to the cervical vertebrae (Haglund 1997a). Depositing loose teeth and isolated mandibles in the cave entrance is an alterative, but seemingly less likely, scenario.

More than one activity or agent is suggested by the osteological profiles, constructed for the different areas within this cave. Evidence for animal transportation of fleshed human body parts to a den at the back of the cave has been identified. The temporary placement of human heads, predominantly of children, teenagers and young adults, in the entrance chamber of this cave is also indicated. There was a lack of evidence to support the theory of whole body burials within the cave. A clear division was identified between outer and inner cave use. The main chamber seems to have formed an arena for human activity, while the passage leading to the back of the cave was dominated by evidence for carnivore scavenging. Whether this differential activity was contemporary, still remains unclear. It has been suggested that the human remains represent Late Neolithic inhumations due to the presence of diagnostic artefacts

(Gilks 1989), but dating by artefact association is problematic in cave environments. Samples of human bone and teeth are currently being radiocarbon dated.

Although human manipulation of cranial material has been identified, the reason for this behaviour remains elusive. Why place heads in a cave chamber, in a fairly inaccessible and hidden location? Caves form a unique environment, processes occurring within then differ from the outside world. Research conducted on the effects of animal remains on cave invertebrate communities produced some interesting results that may provide insight to the interpretation of the activities noted in Raven Scar. Terrell-Nield and MacDonald (1997) noted that small animals placed inside a cave near the entrance became naturally mummified. This transformation or tendency towards desiccation would appear to be due to the variation in temperature and humidity at the threshold area of the cave, with a good flow of air (C Terrell-Nield pers. comm.). This location within the cave may have provided a suitable place to mummify heads. Perhaps those who used Raven Scar cave were aware of these natural processes of transformation and harnessed or manipulated their effects. Artificial and intentional mummification has been a feature of burials from many parts of the world and cultures through time (Aufderheide 2003). Natural processes, once noted, may be manipulated in a specific location or microenvironment to produce the desired effect, and thus be included in the burial regime or ritual. However, the analogy in this instance may be inappropriate. The response of a deceased rat and a human head to specific environmental conditions may not necessarily be similar.

The demography of the cranial material is also of interest. Children are often absent or of minimal representation in the burial record, although they represented a significant proportion of the living population. Due to their reduced representation in death assemblages, interpretations of their life and status in the community are often equally limited in discussions of past societies (Moore & Scott 1997). The placement of a large proportion of children's heads in the cave may represent a deliberate focus on this sector of the community. The death profile may reflect some aspect of their role or value in life, or alternatively, their remains may have had a meaningful role in death.

The significance placed on the cranium during the Iron Age has been highlighted (Green 1998; Ross 1967; Woodward 1992). Head cults, however, need not be restricted to this time period (Wright 1988). There is ethnographic evidence for cranial manipulation after death (Needham 1976) and disassociation of the head from the rest of the body is a recurring feature in the burial record (Harman et al. 1981; Thorpe 2003). Public display is often associated with the removal of the head in past societies, either in the form of trophy collection and exhibition or for the purpose of veneration (Boylston et al. 2000). The hidden and enclosed characteristic of the cave deposition implies an alternative purpose. There are examples of the display or deposition of crania in shrines, sanctuaries and temples, (Mays & Steele 1996; Woodward 1992).The deposition of skulls in Raven Scar Cave may suggest that this special location within the landscape provided a forum for spiritual activity. Green (1998) highlights the characteristics of separation, removal or inaccessibility in defining sacrificial or ritualistic offerings. The deposition of selected human elements in a threshold location may represent such beliefs or intention.

Conclusions

Reanalysis of the human skeletal remains has provided new information relating to the activities occurring in this cave and the surrounding area. The characteristics of the skeletal assemblage highlight a clear distinction between inner and outer cave use. Scavenged human body parts appear to have been brought into the inner passage of the cave by carnivores. Body part representation indicates that exposed corpses in the vicinity were scavenged by animals using this cave as a den. The skeletal remains in this area of the cave represented a minimum number of four individuals, including adult and subadult bones, many exhibited evidence of carnivore chewing. Cranial material dominated the skeletal assemblage from the outer main chamber, representing a minimum number of 15 individuals. It would appear from the evidence that human heads were deliberately placed in the cave; the majority of these only remained for a certain period of time and were then removed, leaving behind the teeth that had become detached from their sockets. The previous interpretation, that this cave site represented a burial area for more than twenty individuals interred in stone cists, now appears doubtful.

It seems unlikely that there will be one unifying explanation of cave use with regard to human deposition. Past perceptions of these locations and their function may have been both fluid and multifaceted. Restoring the human remains back into their context and analysing both the taphonomic and anthropological data in tandem has generated new insight into past activities in these subterranean environments. Actions in the past, however, may not always fall into our modern spectrum of acceptable behaviour. It is clear from the evidence that this location was not simply a repository for burial. The cave's function and relationship with other features in the landscape may have been complex and significant.

Acknowledgements

I would like to thank Tom Lord for providing access to the skeletal material and paper archive. His theories, discussions and general background information relating to this site and others in the locality have been invaluable.

Literature Cited

Aufderheide AC (2003) *The Scientific Study of Mummies.* Cambridge: Cambridge University Press.

Bass WM (1987) *Human Osteology: A Laboratory and field manual.* 4th ed. Special Publication No. 2 of the Missouri Archaeological Society Columbia.

Behrensmeyer AK (1978) Taphonomic and ecological information from bone weathering. *Paleobiology* 4: 150-162.

Bonsall C and Tolan-Smith C (1997) *The Human Use of Caves.* BAR International Series 667 Oxford: BAR Publishing.

Boylston A, Knusel C J, Roberts CA and Dawson M (2000) Investigation of a Romano-British Rural Ritual in Bedford, England. *Journal of Archaeological Science* 27: 241-254.

Bradley R (2000) *An Archaeology of Natural Places.* London: Routledge.

Brothwell DR (1981) *Digging Up Bones: the excavation, treatment and study of human remains.* 3rd ed. London: British Museum.

Buikstra JE and Ubelaker DH (1994) *Standards for data collection from human skeletal remains. Proceedings of a seminar at The Field Museum of Natural History.* Arkansas archaeological survey research series No. 44. Fayetteville, Arkansas: Arkansas Archaeological Survey.

Chamberlain AT (1994) *Human Remains.* London: British Museum Press.

Chamberlain AT (1997) In this dark cavern thy burying place. *British Archaeology* 26.

Dawkins WB (1874) *Cave Hunting: Researches on the Evidence of Caves Respecting the Early Inhabitants of Europe.* London: Macmillian & Co.

Fitton EP and Mitchell D (1950) The Ryedale Windypits. *Cave Science* 2 (12): 162-184.

Gilks JA (1976) Excavations in a cave on Raven Scar, Ingleton, 1973-5. *Transactions British Cave Research Association.* 3 (2): 95-99.

Gilks JA (1985) A bone whistle from Raven Scar Cave North Yorkshire. *Antiquity* 59: 124-5.

Gilks JA (1988) The Cave Burial Research Project. *British Archaeology* 6: 6-7.

Gilks JA (1989) Cave Burials in Northern England. *British Archaeology* 11: 11-15.

Green M (1998) Humans as ritual victims in the later prehistory of Western Europe. *Oxford Journal of Archaeology* 17: 169-189.

Haglund WD (1997a) Dogs and Coyotes: Postmortem Involvement with Human Remains. In WD Haglund and M H Sorg (eds.): *Forensic Taphonomy: The Postmortem Fate of Human Remains.* London: CRC Press; 367-381.

Haglund WD (1997b) Scattered Skeletal Human Remains: Search Strategy Considerations for Locating Missing Teeth. In WD Haglund and MH Sorg (eds.): *Forensic Taphonomy: The Postmortem Fate of Human Remains.* London: CRC Press; 383-394.

Haglund WD, Reay DT and Swindler DR (1989) Canid Scavenging / Disarticulation Sequence of Human Remains in the Pacific Northwest. *Journal of Forensic Sciences* 34 (3): 587-606.

Harman M, Molleson TI, and Price JL (1981) Burials, Bodies and Beheadings in Romano-British and Anglo-Saxon cemeteries. *Bulletin British Museum of Natural History (Geology)* 35 (3): 145-188

Hoffman JM (1979) Age estimations from diaphyseal lengths: two months to twelve years. *Journal Forensic Sciences* 24: 461-469.

King MP (2001) Life and Death in the 'Neolithic': Dwelling-scapes in southern Britain. *European Journal of Archaeology* 4 (3):323-345.

Krogman WM and Iscan MY (1986) *The Human Skeleton in Forensic Medicine.* 2nd ed. Springfield, Illinois: Charles C. Thomas.

Larsen C S (1997) *Bioarchaeology: Interpreting behaviour from the human skeleton.* Cambridge Studies in Biological Anthropology 21 Cambridge: Cambridge University Press.

Lovell NC (1997) Trauma Analysis in Paleopathology. *Yearbook of Physical Anthropology* 40: 130-170.

Lyman RL (1994) *Vertebrate Taphonomy.* Cambridge Manuals in Archaeology. Cambridge: Cambridge University Press.

Mays S and Steele J (1996) A mutilated human skull from Roman St Albans, Hertfordshire, England. *Antiquity* 70: 155-161.

McKern T and Stewart TD (1957) *Skeletal Age Changes in Young American Males, Analyzed from the Standpoint of Identification.* Technical Report EP-Natick.

Massachusetts: Quartermaster Research and Development Command.

Moore J and Scott E (1997) *Invisible People and Processes: Writing Gender and Childhood into European Archaeology.* London: Leicester University Press.

Moorees CFA, Fanning EA and Hunt EE (1963a) Formation and Resorption of Three Deciduous Teeth in Children. *American Journal of Physical Anthropology* 21: 205-213.

Moorees CFA, Fanning EA and Hunt EE (1963b) Age Formation by Stages for Ten Permanent Teeth. *Journal of Dental Research* 42: 1490-1502.

Needham R (1976) Skulls and Causality. *Man* 11: 71-88.

Ross A (1967) *Pagan Celtic Britain.* London: Cardinal/ Sphere.

Scheuer JL, Musgrove JM, and Evans SP (1980) The Estimation of Late Foetal and Perinatal Age from Limb Bone Length by Linear and Logarithmic Regression. *Annals of Human Biology* 7: 257-265.

Simpson E (1950) The Kelcow Caves, Giggleswick, Yorkshire. *Cave Science* 2: 258-62.

Smith BH (1991) Standards of Human Tooth Formation and Dental Age Assessment. In MA Kelly and CS Larsen: *Advances in Dental Anthropology.* New York: Wiley-Liss

Smith BH (1984) Patterns of Molar Wear in Hunter-Gatherers and Agriculturalists. *American Journal of Physical Anthropology* 63: 39-56.

Smith HE. (1865) The Limestone Caves of Craven and their Ancient Inhabitants. *Transactions of the Historical Society of Lancashire and Cheshire* 5: 199-230.

Suchey JM, Owings PA, Wiseley DV and Noguchi TT (1984) Skeletal Aging of Unidentified Persons. In TA Rathbun and JE Buikstra (eds.): *Human Identification: Case Studies in Forensic Anthropology.* Springfield, Illinois: Charles C Thomas.

Terrell-Nield C and MacDonald J (1997) The effects of decomposing animal remains on cave invertebrate communities. *Cave and Karst Science* 24 (2):53-63.

Thorpe N (2003) Anthropology, archaeology, and the origin of warfare. *World Archaeology* 35 (1): 145-165.

Ubelaker DH (1989) The Estimation of Age at Death from Immature Human Bone. In MY Iscan (ed.): *Age Markers in the Human Skeleton.* Springfield, Illinois: Charles C Thomas.

Villa P and Mahieu E (1991) Breakage patterns of human long bones. *Journal of Human Evolution* 21: 27-48.

Woodward A (1992) *Shrines and Sacrifice*. London: BT Batsford ltd/English Heritage.

Wright GRH (1988) The severed head in earliest Neolithic times. *Journal of Prehistoric Religion* 2: 51-56.

A Study of Paget's Disease at Norton Priory, Cheshire.
A Medieval Religious House

Paget's disease at Norton Priory

Anthea Boylston* and Alan Ogden

Biological Anthropology Research Centre
Department of Archaeological Sciences
University of Bradford
Bradford
BD7 1DP
* e-mail address for correspondence: A.Boylston@bradford.ac.uk

Abstract

Norton Priory was established at Runcorn in Cheshire in 1115 AD during the reign of Henry I. It was a medieval religious house whose inhabitants were canons following the rule of St Augustine. Most of the 130 burials excavated during the 1970s were those of older males; a few were elderly females who, perhaps as benefactresses of the establishment, had the right to be buried within the church precinct. Six of the males showed evidence of Paget's disease which, incidentally, is more common in this part of England in the present day than it is in any other part of the country. Paget's disease is a disorder of bone metabolism and affects between 750,000 and 1,000,000 people over 50 in the UK today, involving most commonly the skull, spine, pelvis or femora. The cases from Norton Priory are described and the aetiology of the disease is discussed. In addition, this study includes probably the first description of osteosarcoma in a palaeopathological case of Paget's disease.

Keywords: Paget's disease, osteosarcoma, palaeopathology, Norton Priory, monasticism

Introduction

The earliest definitive study of *osteitis deformans* was carried out by Sir James Paget in the latter part of the nineteenth century (Paget 1877) and the disease has remained something of a mystery ever since. Although it is the second most common bone disease suffered by the elderly after osteoporosis (Morales-Piga et al. 2002), many people are unaware of its existence and the medical establishment is still uncertain of its cause. Unlike osteoporosis, however, the skeleton is patchily affected – in some cases only one skeletal element is affected, but more often Paget's is seen in several elements (Resnick & Niwayama 1988). Moreover, it is not necessarily symmetrical in its distribution; one side of the pelvic or pectoral girdle may be involved but not the other. If the condition is mild, the patient may not be greatly inconvenienced. However, if it is severe, the disease can cause considerable pain and disabilities such as deafness may arise. Where the cranium is involved, the person may become aware that their hat - or even their dentures - no longer fit properly (Fisher 1990).

The mechanism of the disease is one of increased bone turnover. Three phases have been distinguished: an osteoclastic phase where bone is removed and this process can be seen on radiographs as large areas with little bone substance within the cortex. Then there is a quiescent stage followed by chaotic bone-forming activity. "The disease is characterised by anarchic bone remodelling associated with morphological and functional abnormalities of osteoclasts" (Rousiere et al. 2003: 1019). This remodelling produces an enlarged bone that is soft and of poor quality. Macroscopically, such bones appear more porous than normal and are also heavier than their unaffected pair. Radiographic analysis shows a characteristic cotton wool appearance with a distinct line between affected and unaffected parts of the bone. Ideally, histological examination should also be carried out to detect the mosaic pattern of the cement lines but, as this is destructive, it is not always possible.

Pagetic bones are susceptible to invasion by tumour; hence osteosarcoma is a not uncommon complication, as found in one of Sir James Paget's original patients. Pathological fracture may occur or osteoarthritis develop in joints that no longer fit properly.

Amongst the many causes of the disease which have been considered are viruses and environmental or genetic factors. Viruses which have been thought to be implicated are paramyxoviruses, such as measles or canine distemper virus. The latter supposition has led to a debate about whether people might have contracted the disease from their pets (for discussion see Rogers et al. 2002). Some authors have reported several cases of Paget's disease within the same family (Jones & Reed 1967; Rast & Parkes Weber 1937; Aschner et al. 1952). Indeed, Kanis (1991) reported 40 affected members of the same family over five generations. Paget originally viewed the disease as an inflammatory disorder and some patients have noted an improvement after treatment with anti-inflammatories (Resnick & Niwayama 1988).

The geographical distribution of Paget's disease is interesting: it is most common in Britain and rather less frequent in North America, Australia and parts of western Europe (Barker 1981). By contrast, it is almost unknown in Scandinavia, Asia and in native American populations. Barker et al. (1977) carried out an epidemiological study of Paget's disease in fourteen British towns and discovered that the highest prevalence (6.3-8.3%) occurred in Bolton, Preston and Blackburn, all situated in Lancashire. This study was later extended to cover 31 towns (Barker et al. 1980) and an overall prevalence of 3 – 4% in those over the age of 40 was noted, with more men than women being affected. Since then, a decline in the number of people with the disease in England and Wales has been reported (Cooper et al. 1999; van Staa et al. 2002). In other countries, such as Spain, a decrease in its severity has become apparent in recent years (Cundy et al. 1997; Morales-Piga et al. 2002). There has also been an alteration in the distribution of affected elements (Kanis 1991).

Materials and Methods

Norton Priory is situated in the north-west of England near Liverpool on the south bank of the Mersey. In its heyday, the priory held the title to many lands on both sides of the estuary (Greene 1989). It was founded in 1134 by William Fitznigel, the second Baron Halton. The first house was established at Runcorn in 1115 by Augustinian canons from Bridlington but shortly afterwards moved to its present rural location at Norton (Midmer 1979). The Augustinian canons were priest-monks who lived in a monastic setting but were not isolated from the world. Their involvement in the parish was considerable and they had powers to appoint the local clergy (Burton 1994). Undoubtedly most of the burials at Norton Priory were those of the brethren. However, it was the custom at the period for the aristocracy to ensure the survival of their souls by sponsoring religious institutions in order that they could eventually be buried there. Indeed, this kind of sponsorship provided an important source of funding which the monks found hard to resist (Coppack 1990).

After 1300 AD the main patrons of the priory were the Dutton family and three of their wills express the wish to be buried in the lady chapel at Norton. This chapel has been identified by Patrick Greene (1989), who carried out the excavation of the priory foundations. The north-east chapel was constructed during the first half of the thirteenth century. An extension was added to this chapel from the 14th century onwards and the 1978 excavation (the last year in which burials were recovered) revealed a number of burials of individuals of both sexes and children in this area (see Fig. 1).

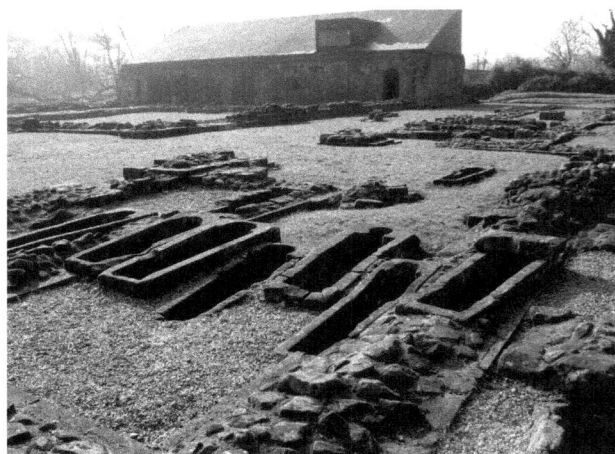

Figure 1. Norton Priory from the north-east. In the foreground are some of the sandstone coffins revealed by the excavation. (Photograph: Darlene Weston).

The excavations resulted in the disinterment of 130 discrete burials which were all very closely dated. Subsequent publication of the site concentrated mainly on the architecture of the building and no analysis of the human remains was included at that time. However, a considerable amount of research did take place in the Department of Anatomy at Liverpool University and six cases of Paget's disease were noted (Connolly, pers comm.), in addition to one individual with leprosy and one or more with tuberculosis.

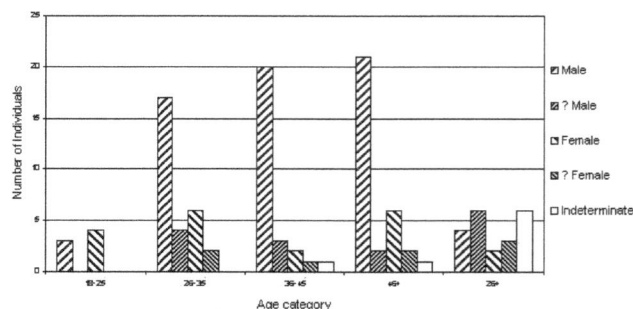

Figure 2. Demography of the adults from Norton Priory.

In 2002, funding became available for a comprehensive demographic and pathological analysis of these burials which was completed at Bradford University. Skeletal analysis was carried out by the first author with the dental analysis and much of the photography being undertaken by the second author. Features described in Bass (1987) and the tables published in Buikstra and Ubelaker (1994) were used to assist in determining the sex of each adult individual. Age estimation was accomplished by using as many methods as possible including dental attrition (Brothwell 1981), pubic symphyseal morphology (Brooks & Suchey 1990), sternal rib ends (Iscan et al. 1984, 1985) and auricular surface changes (Lovejoy et al. 1985).

Table 1: Demographic profile of individuals with Paget's disease

no.	Age	Location	Date of burial	Coffin type	Other conditions
21	Old adult	Centre of nave next to screen	Mid-13th century	Stone (with family crest)	
28	Old adult	Chancel	Late 14th century	Built into wall of chancel	DISH and osteosarcoma
34	Old adult	North-east chapel	Early 14th century	Stone	
50	Old adult (50 yrs plus)	North-east chapel	Late 14th century	None	Complete *spina bifida occulta* of sacrum
53	Old adult	North-east chapel	Early 14th century	Stone	
116	Old adult	West end of nave	15th century	None	Avulsion fracture of medial epicondyle

Table 2: Elements affected by Paget's disease

no	Cranium	Clavicle	Scapula	Spine	Humerus	Ribs	Pelvis	Femur	Tibia
21	✓	B	B	✓	R	✓	R, S	B	
28						✓	L		
34							L		
50		L	L				L, S	R	
53		L	L	✓			L, S	L	L
116	✓			✓	B		B, S	B	B

Where L= Left, R = Right, ✓ = present (side not applicable), B=both L and R elements, and S = Sacrum

The demography of the individuals recovered during excavation is typical for a monastic site (Fig. 2). There were a total of 81 male but only 28 female burials, the latter being situated almost exclusively in the N.E. and eastern Chapels (see Fig. 1) and beneath the north aisle. A mere 13 burials of children were recovered, including one foetus, in the abdomen of burial 135. Eight adults were of indeterminate sex owing to poor preservation of the remains. Age categories include a group where all the epiphyses were fused but no other indications of age were discernible. These are categorised as '26+'.

Results

Six elderly males showed evidence of Paget's disease affecting one or more bones. Their demographic profile and location in the priory church are described in Table 1.

Table 2 and Figure 3 show the distribution of the condition on their skeletons. Almost every case presented unusual aspects, and are summarised below.

Burial 21: This is in many ways the most interesting case of Paget's disease in this group of six individuals. This individual had a highly prestigious burial in a coffin adorned with a family crest. By process of deduction, it is likely that the individual was Roger, brother of the third Baron Halton. This may indicate the familial nature of the disease (discussed later). His coffin was found in an undisturbed condition and preservation of all the skeletal elements was consequently assured. Importantly, his coffin could be dated to the mid-thirteenth century, demonstrating that the disease was present from an early phase in the use of the priory church for burial.

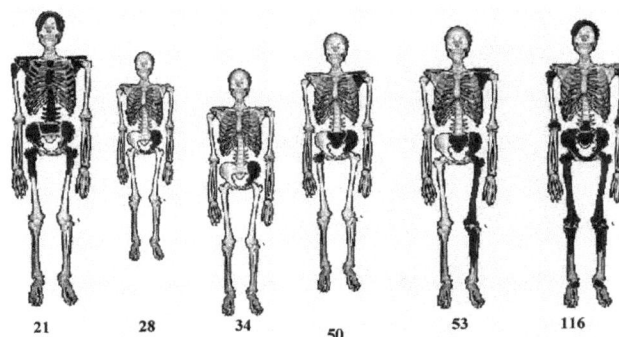

Figure 3. Distribution of bones affected by Paget's disease on the individual skeletons.

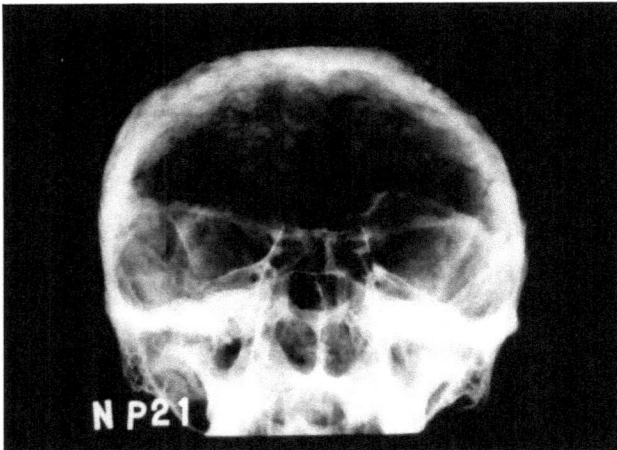

Figure 4. Typical 'cottonwool' appearance of pagetic bone on X-ray (Grave 21).

The frontal bone has been destroyed and hence both the gross thickening of the cranial vault and the deep etching of passages for the middle meningeal arteries on the inner table of the skull are clearly visible. These are characteristic features of Paget's disease. The X-ray of the cranium shows the typical cotton wool appearance produced by this condition (Fig. 4). As the base of the skull was unaffected, it is probable that he had not suffered from deafness or any of the other conditions brought about by nerve impingement. The pectoral girdle was very porous in appearance and the clavicles and scapulae are greatly thickened. Unusually, the right proximal humerus was involved in the disease process with thickening of its articular surface. The entire rib cage, including the manubrium and sternum, was much more porous than normal and the thoracic and lumbar vertebrae were of poor quality and a biscuit-like consistency with the classic 'picture frame' appearance on X-ray (Fig. 5).

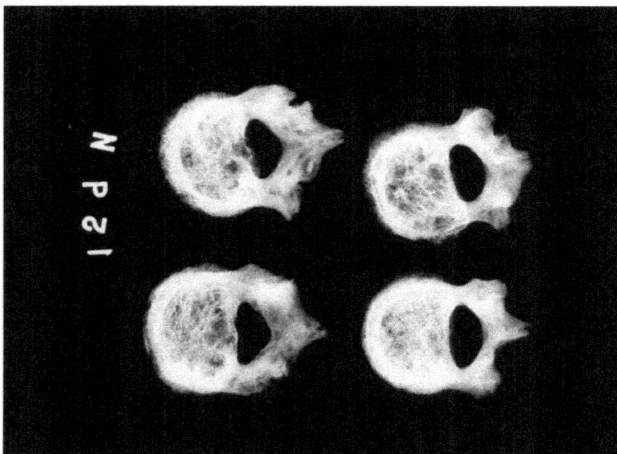

Figure 5. X-ray of vertebrae showing the typical 'picture-frame' appearance (Grave 21).

The sacrum was porous and greatly thickened and the pelvic bones were more severely affected on the right side than the left. Both proximal femora were thickened although their articular surfaces were not affected. The right shoulder joint had adapted to the enlarged humeral head.

Burial 28: The left pelvic bone and both pubic bones were severely affected by the disease with deposition of bone in the iliac fossa, and one rib fragment showed evidence of increased porosity. The left iliac fossa was filled with bony deposition which was quite different from the Pagetic bone (Fig. 6). It had a 'sunburst' appearance and fitted Ragsdale's (1993) criteria for neoplastic invasion of the diseased bony substance. There were patches of similar new bone affecting both sides of the right innominate. The most likely scenario is one of osteosarcoma complicating Paget's disease of the pelvis. This individual also showed evidence of DISH with fusion of the 4th - 11th thoracic vertebrae and widespread ossification at the ligamentous insertions, e.g. on the patellae, the sternum and the pelvis. Additionally, he had osteoarthritis of the left acromioclavicular joint.

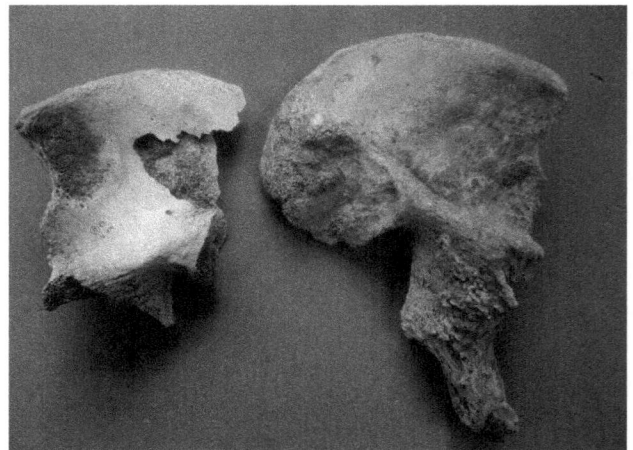

Figure 6 Pelvis of individual from Grave 28 showing early 'sunburst' appearance suggestive of invasion of pagetic bone by osteosarcoma. The highly abnormal bone also affects the right innominate (arrow).

Burial 34: Scanty but definitive evidence of *osteitis deformans* was seen in the left innominate bone.

Burial 50: This individual was mislabelled 52 on the photograph, according to the excavator's notes, and was sent for examination in the laboratory under that guise. On examination of the plans and photographs, it became evident that this number could not be correct as grave 52 was that of an infant. The dentition of this adult burial matched a partial dentition in box 50. This is an important identification as Grave 50 is situated in the north-east chapel where the patronal family members were buried (see Fig. 1).

The disease affected the left side of the pectoral girdle and the left innominate, although in the latter it appeared to be at an early stage. The sacrum was much heavier than normal and replaced by disorganised new bone with the additional complication of complete *spina bifida occulta*. None of the neural arches were fused at the apex. Other conditions affecting this individual were osteoarthritis of the acromioclavicular joints of the shoulder, the spine, right wrist and joints of the left large toe. There are also many enthesopathies, suggesting an active lifestyle.

Burial 53: This grave was so close to burial 50 that their graves intercut each other. Much of the left side of the body was affected by Paget's disease, including the left clavicle, scapula, pelvic bone, proximal femur and tibia. In addition the sacrum, fifth lumbar vertebra and one right rib were affected. Much of the spine was missing but the 11th and 12th thoracic vertebrae were fused.

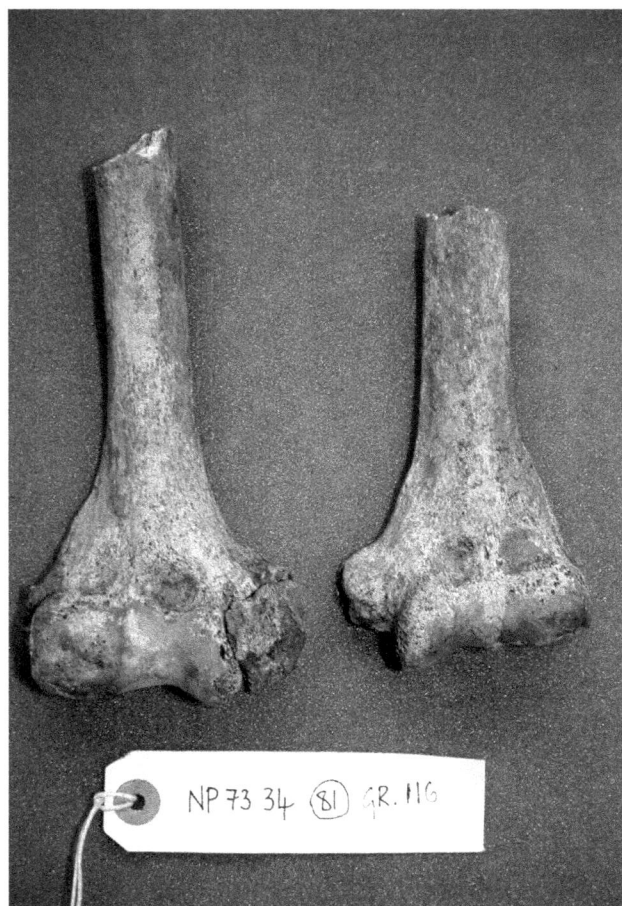

Figure 7. Medial epicondylar avulsion fracture of the right elbow (Grave 116).

Burial 116: This individual was almost as severely affected by Paget's disease as burial 21. There was porous new bone on the inner table of the cranial vault in the midline and ragged deposits on the internal aspect of the frontal bone. The left lateral clavicle and scapula were affected as were the left distal and right proximal and distal humeri. Both pelvic bones and the sacrum had been entirely replaced by porous, disorganised bone, as had both femora and the fifth and sixth lumbar vertebrae. Most of the spine was involved to a lesser degree. The left tibia and proximal right tibia also showed evidence of the disease. On X-ray, a sharp demarcation line was seen between the abnormal and normal bone of the right tibia.

The distortion in shape of the right shoulder had led to impingement of the right humeral head on the acromion and there was osteoarthritis of the right elbow secondary to an avulsion fracture of the medial epicondyle, an injury that probably happened in adolescence (Fig. 7). The joint surface of the right elbow was much larger than the left and on X-ray the cortical bone of the right arm was considerably thicker. The X-ray also showed how severely diseased the right shoulder was by active Paget's disease. The right hip showed signs of osteoarthritis with cystic spaces beneath the articular surface in the midst of the pagetic bone.

Discussion

These cases of Paget's disease are particularly interesting because they span the complete time that the priory church was in use for burial - from the earliest case (Grave 21), dating to the middle of the thirteenth century, to Grave 116, in the fifteenth century. The proximity of Norton Priory to the present-day hotspots of the disease in Lancashire is also fascinating but is difficult to explain. Indeed, since the identification of the 'Lancashire focus' in 1980 (Barker et al. 1980) no convincing explanation has been proposed for this concentration of cases in the north-west of England. Attention has focused on the cotton industry and possible arsenic poisoning related to processing of this commodity (Lever 2002), which would not have been a factor in the medieval period. In any case, this is not a generally accepted theory for the cause of Paget's disease. The interaction between genetic and environmental factors in the disease is, at any event, poorly understood (Kanis 1991).

The location of three of the six burials in the N.E. Chapels (Fig 1) is significant, as we know that the individual with the most severe case of Paget's disease (burial 21) was a member of the Halton family. Burials 50 and 53 were also found in this area, suggesting that the cases of Paget's disease at Norton Priory were not those of the brethren but were more likely to be members of the patronal families, the Duttons and the Haltons. It would suggest that there is a genetic element in these particular cases of Paget's disease. This would seem promising as studies have identified a heritable element to the disease. Kanis's (1991) Sheffield study found evidence for a familial association in 20% of patients in a similar type of *osteitis deformans* to Paget's disease. He also detected a significant increase in the frequency of HLA A9 and B15 in his patients with the familial variant of Paget's disease. Moreover, recent advances in human genome research have suggested that a mutation on a single gene on chromosome 5 may be implicated (Cornelis 2003). Patients with the familial form of Paget's are also likely to have a number of skeletal elements affected and the cases from Norton Priory certainly fall into this category.

Each of these six cases of Paget's, apart from one (burial 34), affected several parts of the skeleton in the classic pattern described by Schmorl (cited in Hamdy 1981). Schmorl noted that the sacrum and lower spine are most likely to be affected by Paget's disease, in contrast to the general perception which is of enlarged heads and limb bones as these manifestations are more visible to both patient and clinician. At Norton Priory the highest prevalence rates were found in the left pelvic bone and sacrum, followed by the left clavicle and scapula (Table 3).

Table 3: Prevalence rates for Paget's disease in individual skeletal elements

Element	N	% of total	% elements from those 45+ years
Sacrum	4	5.5	23.5
Rib	2	2.3	10.5
Cranium	2	1.9	8.3
R scapula	1	1.4	9.1
L scapula	3	4.5	12.5
R clavicle	1	1.8	4.5
L clavicle	3	5.3	12.5
R humerus	2	3.2	8.0
L humerus	1	1.6	3.4
R innominate	2	2.3	9.1
L innominate	5	5.8	21.7
R femur	3	4.5	12.0
L femur	3	4.3	12.0
R tibia	1	1.7	4.5
L tibia	2	3.4	8.3

Some of those with Paget's disease also presented other interesting and unusual features. Notable amongst these was the invasion by tumour bone of the abnormal bone of the pelvis of burial 28. Osteosarcoma was recognised by Sir James Paget as one quite frequent consequence of bone abnormalities caused by the disease. This has not been described in an archaeological case before now. The cancerous bone is quite distinct from the pagetic tissue that it invaded.

Equally interesting is the individual from Grave 116. In addition to widespread Paget's disease and secondary osteoarthritis of the hip, he exhibited an unusual healed but ununited fracture of the elbow. The discrepancy in size between the articular surfaces of his two elbows and the fact that the right epicondyle had been separated from the rest of the bone suggest that some activity took place in adolescence and affected the right elbow preferentially. It seems highly probable that this individual was a knight who was training in medieval combat from an early age. This injury has been found in a battle victim who was killed at the Battle of Towton in AD 1461 (Knüsel 2000) but on this occasion it occurred in the left elbow. A third individual with Paget's disease (Grave 50) also had *spina bifida occulta* in a sacrum which was completely replaced by abnormal bone.

The most ancient evidence for the disease in England dates to the late Anglo-Saxon period. Wells and Woodhouse (1975) reported a case from Jarrow Monastery with the classic radiological appearances and there have been several individuals with Paget's reported from Winchester at around the same period (Price 1975).

One of the few other sites where more than one or two individuals with Paget's disease have been recorded palaeopathologically is St Mary Grace's Priory in London, on the site of the Royal Mint (Waldron 1992). Here 14 of over 700 adults showed evidence of the condition, although in some it was more subtle than in others and was only discovered on X-ray. The pattern here was similar to that seen at Norton Priory with the greatest degree of involvement being found in the pelvis. Waldron calculated an overall prevalence of 3% of males and 4% of females. The rate at Norton Priory was 5% of all adults but 19% of those aged over 45 years. This is an extraordinarily high figure by any standards and suggests that there is something unusual about the burials in this church precinct. A further comparison is provided by a very comprehensive study by Rogers and co-workers of 2770 individuals buried in the churchyard of St Peter's, Barton-on-Humber, Lincolnshire (Rogers et al. 2002). They found a more normal prevalence before 1500 AD of 1.7% and post-1500 AD of 3.1% in those aged over 40 years at death. Preliminary work on 10,417 individuals from Spitalfields Market, London (Connell 2002) has revealed at least eight cases of Paget's disease and no doubt considerably more will be forthcoming once the complete assemblage is studied in detail.

There is no doubt that the six cases of Paget's disease from Norton Priory form a major addition to the history of the disease in Britain. They were found in a part of the country which, even in modern times, has an unusually high incidence of this condition. However, despite the huge amount of research that has been carried out up to the present time, it has not been possible to detect environmental or other factors that are applicable to the north-west of England but not to be found in parts of the world where Paget's disease is rare.

Acknowledgements

The authors would like to acknowledge the enormous assistance they have received from Lynn Smith, Joanne Brown and Steven Miller on the curatorial staff at Norton Priory, from Bob Connolly at Liverpool University, and from Darlene Weston (preparing figures) and Chris Knüsel (commenting upon an earlier draft). The Trustees of the Norton Priory Museum and Gardens are thanked for their support and encouragement. Chris Howard-Davis and Alison Plummer of Oxford Archaeology North are thanked for initiating the re-examination of the Norton Priory human remains. Funding was provided by English Heritage.

Literature Cited

Aschner BM, Hurst LA and Roizin L (1952) A genetic study of Paget's disease (*osteitis deformans*) in monozygotic twin brothers. *Acta Geneticae Medicae et Gemmelologiae* 1: 67-79.

Barker DJP (1981) The epidemiology of Paget's disease. *Metabolic Bone Disease-related Research* 4: 231-4.

Barker DJP, Clough PWL, Guyer PB, and Gardner MJ (1977) Paget's disease of bone in 14 British towns. *British Medical Journal* i: 1181-3.

Barker DJP, Chamberlain AT, Guyer PB and Gardner MU (1980) Paget's disease of bone: the Lancashire focus. *British Medical Journal* 280: 1105-7.

Bass WM (1987) *Human Osteology: a Laboratory and Field Manual.* Missouri: Missouri Archaeological Society.

Brooks S and Suchey J (1990) Skeletal age determination based on the os pubis: a comparison of the Acsadi-Nemeskeri and Suchey-Brooks methods. *Human Evolution* 5: 227-38.

Brothwell DR (1981) *Digging up Bones.* 3rd edition. London: British Museum (Natural History).

Buikstra JE and Ubelaker DH (eds) (1994) *Standards for Data Collection from Human Skeletal Remains.* Fayetteville: Arkansas Archaeological Survey Research Series, no. 44.

Burton J (1994) *Monastic and Religious Orders in Britain 1000 – 1300.* Cambridge: Cambridge University Press.

Connell B (2002) *The Cemetery Population from Spitalfields Market, London: an Osteological Pilot Study and Post-excavation Assessment.* Unpublished bone report. Museum of London Specialist Services.

Cooper C, Schafheutle K, Dennison E, Kellingray S, Guyer P, and Barker D (1999) The epidemiology of Paget's disease in Britain: is the prevalence decreasing? *Journal of Bone and Mineral Research* 14: 192-7.

Coppack G (1990) *Abbeys and Priories.* London: BT Batsford.

Cornelis F (2003) Genetics and clinical practice in rheumatology. *Joint Bone Spine* 70: 458-64.

Cundy T, McAnulty K, Wattie G, Gamble G, Rutland M, and Ibbertson HK (1997) Evidence for secular change in Paget's disease. *Bone* 20: 69-71.

Fisher EW (1990) Rhinological manifestations of Paget's disease of bone (osteitis deformans). *Journal of Cranio-Maxillo-Facial Surgery* 18: 169-72.

Greene P (1989) *Norton Priory: the Archaeology of a Medieval Religious House.* Cambridge: Cambridge University Press.

Hamdy RC (1981) *Paget's Disease of Bone: Assessment and Management.* Eastbourne: Armour Pharmaceutical.

Iscan MY, Loth SR, and Wright RK (1984) Age estimation from the rib by phase analysis: white males. *Journal of Forensic Science* 29: 1094-1104.

Iscan MY, Loth SR, and Wright RK (1985) Age estimation from the rib by phase analysis: white females. *Journal of Forensic Science* 30: 853-63.

Jones JV and Reed MF (1967) Paget's disease: family with six cases. *British Medical Journal* 4: 90-1.

Kanis JA (1991) *Pathophysiology and Treatment of Paget's Disease of Bone.* London: Martin Dunitz.

Knüsel C (2000) Activity-related skeletal change. In V Fiorato, A Boylston, and C Knusel (eds): *Blood red roses: the archaeology of a mass grave from the Battle of Towton AD 1461.* Oxford: Oxbow Books; 103-18

Lever JH (2002) Paget's disease of bone in Lancashire and arsenic pesticide in cotton mill wastewater: a speculative hypothesis. *Bone* 31: 434-6.

Lovejoy CO, Meindl S, Przybeck TR, and Mensforth BP (1985) Chronological metamorphosis of the auricular surface of the ilium. A new method for the determination of adult skeletal age at death. *American Journal of Physical Anthropology* 68: 15-28.

Midmer R. (1979) *English Mediaeval Monasteries 1066-1540: a Summary.* London: Heinemann.

Morales-Piga AA, Bachiller-Corral FJ, Abraira V, Beltran J, and Rapado A (2002) Is clinical expressiveness of Paget's disease of bone decreasing? *Bone* 30: 399-403.

Paget J (1877) On a form of chronic inflammation of bones (osteitis deformans). *Medico-chirurgical Transactions*, London 60: 37-63.

Price JL (1975) The radiology of excavated Saxon and medieval human remains from Winchester. *Clin Radiol* 26: 363-70.

Ragsdale BD (1993) Morphologic analysis of skeletal lesions: correlation of imaging studies and pathologic findings. *Advances in Pathology and Laboratory Medicine* 6: 445-90.

Rast H and Parkes Weber F (1937) Paget's bone disease in three sisters. *British Medical Journal* i: 918.

Resnick D and Niwayama G (1988) *Diagnosis of Bone and Joint Disorders.* 2nd edition. Philadelphia: WB Saunders Company.

Rogers J, Jeffrey DR and Watt I (2002) Paget's disease in an archeological population. *Journal of Bone and Mineral Research* 17: 1127-34.

Rousiere M, Michou L, Cornelis F and Orcel P. (2003) Paget's disease of bone. *Best Practice and Research in Clinical Rheumatology* 17: 1019-41.

Van Staa TP, Selby P, Leufkens HGM, Lyles K, Sprafka JM and Cooper C. (2002) Incidence and natural history of Paget's disease of bone in England and Wales. *Journal of Bone and Mineral Research* 17: 465-71.

Waldron T. (1992) *The Human Remains from the Royal Mint Site. Unpublished bone report.* Museum of London Specialist Services.

Wells C and Woodhouse NJY. (1975) Paget's disease in an Anglo-Saxon. *Medical History* 19: 396-400.

The Bog Bodies of Northwestern Europe: Current Research

Northwestern European Bog Bodies

Heather Gill-Robinson

Department of Anthropology, Fletcher Argue 145, University of Manitoba, Winnipeg, Manitoba
R3C 2N2, Canada

hgrobinson@mts.net

Abstract
Numerous bog bodies, or body parts, have been discovered in acidic peat bogs in northwestern Europe, although very few of these remains are still in existence. Many of the bog bodies have extensive soft tissue including skin, muscle and internal organs. This paper explores some of the current research being conducted with the bog bodies and discusses the Schloss Gottorf Bog Body Research Project, an anthropological re-analysis of a collection of six bog bodies from northern Germany.

Keywords Bog bodies, mummies, imaging, taphonomy, DNA, Germany, Europe

Introduction

The well-preserved human remains recovered from the peat of northwestern Europe are commonly known as bog bodies. Although a few bodies are exceptionally well preserved, other bog bodies may have only partial soft tissue preservation. In alkaline peat, such as can be found in the fens of Norfolk, the bodies are preserved as skeletons with no remaining soft tissue (Healy & Housely 1992). In areas of acidic peat the soft tissue may be exceptionally well preserved, but bone is severely demineralised. In some of these bodies the bones may be so demineralised that the bodies have become flattened skins only a few centimetres thick (Gebühr 2002, Glob 1969, van der Sanden 1996). All bog bodies are spontaneous mummies and had no anthropogenic contribution to their preservation.

Bog bodies can be divided into three groups: those which still exist, those which exist only in records, and finally those which were discovered, but not reported. The first group of bodies represents those whose discoveries were recorded in parish records, local newspapers, antiquarian journals or personal correspondence and which can be traced today, often to museum displays and storerooms. The second group, commonly known as "paper bog bodies" (van der Sanden 1996), refers to those bodies which exist in a written record, but of which there remain no physical traces. Caution must be used when referring to these bodies as facts can no longer be checked for accuracy and the original reports may be erroneous or vague. Potentially the largest group is that of bog bodies that remain unrecorded in any source. Early bog finds were seldom reported and superstitions surrounded these corpses, which were often hastily re-buried (van der Sanden 1996).

The preservation processes in peat bogs have been a matter of speculation since bog bodies have been discovered. In one of the earliest articles to speculate on peat and preservation (Hunt 1866), it was reported that peat was destructive to human remains, although a single preserved specimen discussed in the same article contradicted the author's belief. Another author (Cotton 1960: 247) suggested that the preservation would only result from "a combination of suitable soil conditions and a specialized burial rite." Most theories centre upon the presence of tannins, the anoxic nature of the peat or a combination of these factors (Evershed 1990). Theories relating to a lack of oxygen in the lower levels of peat inhibiting decay were also proposed (Coles 1984, Connolly 1985). Although preservation of soft tissue in peat bogs is generally attributed to the presence of tannic acids (Micozzi 1991), other environmental mechanisms, including an anaerobic aquatic environment, may contribute to the spontaneous preservation of these bodies. Painter (1991a) argued that the so-called tanning of bog body skin is not from vegetable tannins, as commonly believed, as the polyphenols necessary for production of vegetable tannins are absent in *Sphagnum* mosses. Painter's research indicated that sphagnan, an anionic polysaccharide that becomes soluble during the process of breakdown from dead *sphagnum* moss to peat, was responsible for the tanning of bog body skin (Painter 1991a, 1991b, 1995).

Bog body preservation is highly variable. Some bodies will be preserved as soft tissue corpses with highly demineralised bones; others have good soft tissue preservation in some parts and skeletonisation of other body parts, while still others are preserved as "flat bodies", mainly skin with some soft tissue and virtually no skeletal material. These variations seem to be based upon microenvironmental preservation, where minute differences in water levels (Gill-Robinson 1998, 2000, 2001, 2002) and chemical or botanical composition differentially affect the preservation of a corpse crossing several microenvironments.

Are the numbers correct?

Estimates of the number of bog bodies recovered are highly variable and range from "hundreds" (Coles and Coles 1989: 177) up to about 2,000 (Aufderheide 2003; Brothwell and Gill-Robinson 2002; Chamberlain and Parker Pearson 2001), with several estimates between 1,000 and 1,400 (e.g. Brothwell 1996; Fischer 1998; Menon 1997; Parker Pearson 1999). It is likely, however, that the numbers are vastly over-estimated, due, in part, to the research of Dr. Alfred Dieck. Dieck's main catalogue of the bog bodies (1965) listed several bodies that could not be verified. In a later publication, Dieck (1986) estimated 1,850 bog bodies or body parts. Recent research, however, has suggested that many of the bodies listed in Dieck's publications were, in fact, created by Dieck and never existed (Eisenbeiss 1992, 1994, 2003; van der Sanden 1993, 2003). It is impossible to determine how many bog bodies have been discovered, particularly in light of paper bodies and those bodies that were never reported. It is estimated that about 40 bog bodies currently exist in museum storerooms and displays.

One recent research project led to the development of a database listing 369 confirmed bog bodies, including those corroborated by multiple sources although not necessarily still in existence. That research has provided basic demographic and archaeological data about the bodies (Brothwell & Gill-Robinson 2002, Gill-Robinson 2003).

Bog bodies and DNA

During the Lindow research project, attempts were made to collect ancient DNA. Although DNA was successfully obtained from *Escherichia coli* in the gut contents of the Lindow Man remains, no DNA was retrieved from the body itself (Fricker et al. 1997).

In 2002 the Paleo-DNA Laboratory of Lakehead University in Thunder Bay, Canada, successfully extracted and amplified DNA from two Dutch bog bodies. The bodies had been found together and one lay upon the arm of the other. Anthropological investigation determined that both bodies were male. DNA analysis confirmed that not only were both bodies male, but they had no direct maternal association. Tests are currently underway to ascertain whether there is paternal affiliation between the two bodies (Matheson, pers. comm.).

The ability to use DNA analysis in the examination and interpretation of bog bodies is a great advantage. In the case of the adolescent in the Schloss Gottorf collection, the "Windeby Child", traditional methods of skeletal sexing may be impossible. It is well known that accurately sexing children and early adolescents is difficult (Buikstra & Ubelaker 1994: 16; Mays 1998: 38; Saunders 2000; Sutter 2003). The bones of the Windeby Child, like those of all bog bodies, are severely demineralised and distorted and hence any attempt to undertake standard morphometric analyses for sex determination may prove impossible. DNA may thus be an appropriate course of action for this particular case.

Furthermore, the Windeby Child is one of two bodies found only a few metres apart. While AMS radiocarbon dating indicates that the bodies are not contemporary (Gebühr 2002), there may be a familial affiliation that could be determined with DNA. The second body is severely demineralised, however, and it may not be possible for samples suitable for DNA analysis to be extracted.

Recent bog body research projects

Although some of the bog bodies have undergone intensive anthropological investigations, many were examined briefly, conserved and placed on display with no further analyses. It is imperative that the surviving bog bodies be examined using modern techniques and technology in order to gain as much information as possible about these valuable human remains.

There are few projects currently in progress that involve the re-examination of bog bodies. In 1989, Brothwell and colleagues re-examined the Huldremose Woman from Denmark. Scanning Electron Microscopy (SEM) of scalp hair, which had originally been presumed absent, determined that the hair had been shaved very close to the scalp (Brothwell et al. 1990a, 1990b). The X-ray imaging of the body indicated that fractures previously identified as antemortem or perimortem were rather pseudopathologies (Brothwell et al. 1990a, 1990b). Pseudopathologies are lesions suggestive of trauma and palaeopathology, but that can be attributed to taphonomic variables (Wells 1967) and are particularly common in the peat bog bodies of northwestern Europe. The acidic environment of peat bogs leads to severe demineralisation of the skeletal material, particularly when the pressure from the overlying peat is considered, and can cause misinterpretation of fractures and other skeletal lesions (Brothwell & Gill-Robinson 2002). As many of the bog bodies were discovered and excavated during peat cutting processes, it is common for the skin and muscles layers to be damaged. Pieces of limbs may be unintentionally cut or severed when the peat spade is driven through the body prior to its discovery and may lead to interpretation as perimortem trauma.

In a project begun in 1996, Dr. Peter Pieper and colleagues applied forensic anthropological techniques to the re-examination of five bog bodies at the Landesmuseum Natur und Mensch in Oldenburg, Germany (Pieper 2003). During the re-analysis, one body previously reported as an adult female ("Woman from Sedelsberg") was identified as an adolescent male. The body of a male child, Kayhausen Boy, was imaged used Magnetic Resonance Tomography (MRT), allowing the identification of three parallel stab wounds on the neck (Pieper 2003: 110). Additional examination of the same body included the analysis of previously-removed internal organs, palaeodietary reconstruction from gut contents and endoscopy. A third body, an adult male that known as "Red Franz" or the "Neu Versen Man", was also subjected for forensic investigation. The new examination identified a cut throat as the cause of death, as well as healed trauma from a possible arrow injury and the presence of "rider's facets" (Pieper 2003). The adult male body from Husbäke in Germany was recorded in three dimensions through both computed tomography and holography. This project was the first use of holography for a bog body, providing both master holograms of the entire body for archive purposes and display holograms for exhibition (Frey et al. 2003).

In 2000, a team from Denmark began to re-examine the Grauballe Man from the Moesgard Museum in Denmark. The body was subjected to a substantial program of imaging including computed tomography (CT) and facial reconstruction. Results again identified pseudopathologies and revealed aspects of conservation that may have previously affected the interpretation and analysis of the body (Asingh 2003a, 2003b). A programme of CT imaging of the Danish bog bodies is under way; several Danish bog bodies have been scanned and the images are currently being processed and analysed (Lynnerup, pers. comm.).

Experimental archaeology has also been undertaken in order to try to understand the processes of bog body taphonomy (Gill-Robinson 1996, 1998, 2001, 2002; Holmes 2001; Janaway et al. 2003). The first experimental research using animals in peat in an effort to understand the processes of preservation and decomposition were conducted by Ellermann and reported in 1917. Ellermann conducted a series of experiments using rodents and, eventually, human skin placed in peat mixtures in his laboratory. Through this research Ellermann determined that, in acidic peat, bones would demineralise and the skin become leathery. In a neutral peat mixture there was more likely to be preserved skeletal material, but little or no "tanning" of the skin (Ellermann 1917). Although this research was conducted in a laboratory rather in the field, it can be viewed as the first experimental attempt to understand the taphonomic factors affecting bog bodies.

Recent research by Janaway and co-workers has used pigs buried in acidic upland peat in the United Kingdom to determine taphonomy for forensic and archaeological

applications (Janaway et al. 2003). While upland peat is mainly saturated, it can experience variable water levels, including dry periods (Janaway et al. 2003), unlike the raised peat bogs (lowland) where most bog bodies have been found. The work in the upland peat demonstrates that although soft tissue preservation did not reach the level seen in some archaeological bodies from lowland peat, decomposition was still reduced. Soft tissue preserved longer than would be expected in a dry soil burial of comparable depth and time duration (Janaway et al. 2003).

One research project has specifically addressed the taphonomy of lowland raised bog peat as it relates to archaeological human remains through the burial of piglets as human analogues (Gill-Robinson 1996, 1998, 2000, 2001, 2002). Burial of humans or human substitutes in peat was necessary in an attempt to simulate the original burial environments of the ancient bog bodies as closely as was possible, despite the time difference (i.e. 2000 b.p. compared with the present). The purpose of experimental piglet burials was to determine which environmental factors might be responsible for peat bog body preservation. It was shown that higher levels of water at the bog site led to better soft tissue preservation, but that numerous other factors, including micro-environmental variations, contributed to selective preservation of bog bodies (Gill-Robinson 2000, 2002). This research was fairly short-term, the piglets were in the peat for a maximum of three years, and thus needs to be replicated over a longer period of time.

Finally, research also currently in progress is assessing public perceptions of the display of the bog bodies in both Germany (Gebühr, pers. comm.) and Canada (Gill-Robinson, in press). Although bog bodies have been on display in Germany, Denmark, Ireland, England and the Netherlands for decades, few complaints have been received from the general public regarding the display of actual human remains.

In 2003, seven bog bodies were brought to Canada as part of a large exhibition of wetland archaeology entitled "The Mysterious Bog People: Rituals and Sacrifice in Ancient Europe". The exhibition is a joint collaboration between the Drents Museum of Assen in the Netherlands, the Niedersächsisches Landesmuseum of Hanover (Germany), the Canadian Museum of Civilization of Gatineau (Canada) and the Glenbow Museum of Calgary (Canada). Entirely curated in Europe, the exhibition consists of more than 400 artefacts from bog sites in northwestern Europe, as well as the seven preserved ancient bodies. The primary focus of the exhibition is to present the artefacts and bodies as evidence of votive offerings to sacred wetland sites.

Though the same exhibition had run in Hanover, Germany, without incident, less than a week after the exhibition opened at the Museum of Civilization in

Gatineau, it faced sharp criticism for the public display of human remains (Gill-Robinson, in press). While there is no specific legislation restricting or preventing the display of human remains as part of legitimate museum exhibitions, it is generally not an acceptable practice in Canada. The origin of these unwritten ethical guidelines stem from the fact that the First Nations (Native) groups in Canada clearly still exist and many human remains in this country can be directly linked to their living descendents. In many First Nations cultures, it is unacceptable to display human remains. Focus groups that were held in the planning stages for the exhibition included representatives of First Nations groups, to ensure that the exhibition would not be offensive from an Aboriginal cultural perspective (McLeod O'Reilly, pers. comm.; Schmidt 2002). The controversy over the inclusion of the bog bodies in this exhibition stemmed not from First Nations concerns, but other public disapproval of the display of human remains (Gessel 2002). In Canada, there is a great deal of sensitivity about this issue in non-Aboriginal populations, partially through increased awareness of First Nations views towards aspects of archaeology and physical anthropology (Schmidt 2002). Another facet of the issue revolved around not just from the display of the remains, but also from the marketing of souvenirs such as T-shirts and tote bags, which included images of the bog bodies (Gill-Robinson, in press).

The Schloss Gottorf Bog Body Research Project

As discussed above, the need to locate, identify and re-analyse all existing bog bodies is great. One such project, currently in progress, is the Schloss Gottorf Bog Body Research Project. In Schleswig-Holstein, the region in northern Germany from which the Schloss Gottorf bodies originate, cremation was the predominant form of disposal of the dead during the Iron Age (Gebühr 2002). There are very few skeletons from Iron Age Schleswig-Holstein available for analysis; there is, however, a huge amount of cremated bone, much of which is has not been studied. The re-examination of the bog bodies at Schloss Gottorf can potentially provide data related to health, diet and lifestyle in Iron Age northern Germany that is not currently available due, in part, to the limited amount of skeletal material from this region.

More than 60 bodies or body parts, including at least five human mummies have been excavated from the peat of Schleswig-Holstein, northern Germany (von Haugwitz 1993). It is impossible to more precise about the specific number, particularly in light of the issues associated with Alfred Dieck, as discussed above. Five of the mummies, one skull and one mandible are now part of the collection of the Archäologisches Landesmuseum at Schloss Gottorf in Schleswig.

The group of bog bodies at the Archäologisches Landesmuseum is a unique collection as it includes two

of the "flat" bodies with completely demineralised bones, and a potential adolescent female. The group represents about 15% of the locatable bog bodies still in existence and is also the largest collection of bog bodies on permanent display in a single museum. All of the bodies date to the Scandinavian Iron Age, approximately 2,000 years ago (500 B.C. to 800 A.D) (Gebühr 2002; van der Plicht et al. 2004). The mummies display varying levels of soft tissue preservation, but in all cases (except the skull and mandible), extensive soft tissue remains on the bodies.

At the time of excavation, each of the remains was examined, prior to storage or conservation for display, although this information was not extensively published (Aletsee 1967; Asmus 1955a, 1955b; Caselitz 1979; Gebühr 1979; Gruner 1979; Helmer 1983; Ketelsen 1996; Martin 1967; Schiebler & Schaefer 1961; Struve 1967). Only summary information about some of the bodies has been made available in English (Glob 1969; van der Sanden 1996).

All of the bodies will undergo a complete physical re-evaluation. Imaging is a priority for this project, as non-invasive studies are preferred. Both plain film X-rays and CT scanning will be used, depending on the method deemed most appropriate for each individual body. The purpose of the imaging is both diagnostic and reconstructive. Any remaining skeletal material in bog bodies is usually severely demineralised. Imaging, whether through traditional plain film radiography or multi-slice CT (MSCT), provides evidence of the current extent of the skeletal material and an indication of the level of internal preservation of the bodies. Depending upon the quality of bone preservation, trauma or palaeopathology may be visible on the images. Re-examination of previously reported fractures, through both the images and the bones themselves, where possible, may allow more specific interpretation as to whether the fractures were antemortem, perimortem or taphonomic in origin. It may also be possible to visualise internal organs and any evidence of methods used to conserve the bog bodies or prepare them for museum display. In the case of the Grauballe Man of Denmark, for example, it is now known that material was injected into the nose to allow re-formation prior to the display of this body (Asingh 2003b). It is presently not known whether any reconstructive techniques have been used with the bog bodies of Schloss Gottorf.

Through the technology at the Biological Digital Imaging Anthropology Laboratory (BDIAL) at the Department of Anthropology, University of Manitoba, all images of all bodies will be analysed in detail and, where appropriate, computerised reconstruction and rapid prototypes will be produced in three dimensions. These prototypes will allow the visualisation of the skeletal material beneath the skin. Where the fractures are beneath soft tissue, full-scale three-dimensional replicas of the bones can be produced using rapid prototyping, allowing careful examination of both the image and the bone (via the model), to provide the most accurate assessment and interpretation of the fracture.

The skull of the Windeby Child will be laser scanned to produce a white-light hologram, like that seen in the recent project at the Oldenburg Museum (Frey et al. 2003; Pieper 2003). The hologram not only provides a fascinating visual presentation of the skull for museum visitors, it also provides a permanent, full-scale three-dimensional representation of the skull for archival purposes.

Permission has been obtained to undertake DNA analysis of at least one body (Windeby Child) in an attempt to confirm sex. If suitable samples can be extracted the second body from the same site (Windeby II) will also be tested against the Windeby Child for potential familial affiliation.

Other planned analyses include the examination of gut contents or hair samples for palaeoparasites. Samples of hair will also be tested using stable isotope analysis and trace element analysis, in an effort to identify aspects of diet. There are, for example, several large shell middens in the region, all of which date to the Iron Age (Harck 1973). It is possible that the bog bodies had a high marine component to their diet, which would shed new light on a population that is currently believed to have consumed an agrarian terrestrial diet.

Conclusion

The bog bodies of northwest Europe are a unique resource in archaeology and physical anthropology. In general, in the past few decades there has been little new research in the physical analysis of the bog bodies, but new research programmes have been developed for the re-analysis and interpretation of the bog bodies. It is hoped that the advances in mummy imaging, the recent developments in DNA analysis and the current projects to re-examine surviving bog bodies will provide new data and allow even more detailed interpretations of these remarkable human remains.

Acknowledgements

For research support and assistance, the author would like to thank Dr Michael Gebühr and the Archäologisches Landesmuseum (Schloss Gottorf, Schleswig, Germany) and Dr. Carney Matheson of the Paleo-DNA Laboratory (Lakehead University, Thunder Bay, Canada). Research funding was provided byDr. Robert Hoppa, a Duff Roblin Fellowship (University of Manitoba) and the Deutscher Akademischer Austausch Dienst (DAAD). Conference funding was provided by St. John's College (University of Manitoba) and the University of Manitoba Graduate Student Association.

Literature Cited

Aletsee L (1967) Datierungsversuch der Moorleichen-funde von Datgen 1959/60. *Offa* 24:79-83.

Asingh P (2003a) The Grauballe Man. A well-preserved Iron Age bog body. Old and new examinations. In Lynnerup N, Andreasen C and Berglund, J (eds). *Mummies in a New Millenium.* Danish Polar Center: Copenhagen; 50-56.

Asingh P (2003b) Death in the museum. How do we handle the exhibition of a bog body? In N Lynnerup, C Andreasen, and J Berglund (eds): *Mummies in a New Millenium.* Copenhagen: Danish Polar Center; 92-95.

Asmus W (1955a) Auffindung und Bergung der Moorleichen im Großen Moor bei Hunteburg, Kr. Wittlage. *Die Kunde* NF. 6:37-40.

Asmus W (1955b) Der anthropologische Befund der Moorleichen vom Großen Moor bei Hamburg. *Die Kunde* NF 6:50-59.

Aufderheide A (2003) *The Scientific Study of Mummies.* Cambridge: Cambridge University Press.

Brothwell DR (1996) European bog bodies: current state of research and preservation. In K Spindler, H Wilfing, E Rastbichler-Zissernig, D zur Nedden, and H Nothdurfter (eds): *Human Mummies: A Global Survey of their Status and the Techniques of Conservation. The Man in the Ice, Volume 3.* Vienna: Springer Verlag; 161- 172.

Brothwell D and Gill-Robinson HC (2002) Taphonomic and forensic aspects of bog bodies. In W Haglund and M Sorg (eds): *Modern Methods in Forensic Taphonomy.* Boca Raton: CRC Press; 119-132.

Brothwell D, Holden T, Liversage D, Gottleib B, Bennike P, and Boesen, J (1990a) Establishing a minimum damage procedure for the gut sampling of intact human bodies: the case of the Huldremose woman. *Antiquity* 64: 830-835.

Brothwell D, Liversage D and Gottleib B (1990b) Radiographic and forensic aspects of the female Huldremose body. *Journal of Danish Archaeology* 9:157-178.

Buikstra JF and Ubelaker DH (1994) *Standards for Data Collection from Human Skeletal Remains.* Fayetteville: Arkansas Archaeological Survey Research Series No. 44. Arkanas Archaeological Survey

Caselitz P (1979) Aspekte zur Ernahrung in der römischen Kaiserzeit, dargestellt an der Moorleiche von Windeby - I. *Offa* 36:108-115.

Chamberlain AT and Parker Pearson M (2001) *Earthly Remains.* London: British Museum Press.

Coles JM (1984) *The Archaeology Wetlands.* Edinburgh: Edinburgh University Press.

Coles J and Coles B (1989) *People of the Wetlands: Bogs, Bodies and Lake-Dwellers.* London: Thames and Hudson.

Connolly RC (1985) Lindow Man: Britain's prehistoric bog body. *Anthropology Today* 1(5): 15-17.

Cotton MA (1960) Preservation in Iron Age bog burials. *The Archaeological News Letter*: 247-251.

Eisenbeiß S (1992) *Berichte über Moorleichen aus Niedersachsen im Nachlass von Alfred Dieck.* Unpublished Magister Thesis, Universität Hamburg, Germany.

Eisenbeiß S (1994) Berichte über Moorleichen aus Niedersachsen im Nachlaß von Alfred Dieck. *Die Kunde* N.F. 45:91-120.

Eisenbeiß S (2003) Bog-bodies in Lower Saxony – rumours and facts: An analysis of Alfred Dieck's sources of information. In A Bauerochse and H Haßmann (eds): *Peatlands – Archaeological Sites – Archives of Nature – Nature Conservation – Wise Use. Proceedings of the Peatland Conference 2002 in Hannover, Germany.* Rahden, Westf: Verlag Marie Leidorf; 143-150.

Ellermann V (1917) Eine eigentümliche Veräderung von Liechen in Torfmooren ("Moorgerbung"). *Vierteljahr-schrift für ger. Med. und öff. San. – Wesen* 54: 181-192.

Evershed RP (1990) Lipids from samples of skin from seven Dutch bog bodies: preliminary report. *Archaeometry* 12(2): 139-153.

Fischer C (1998) Bog bodies of Denmark and northwestern Europe. In A Cockburn, E Cockburn, and TA Reyman (eds): *Mummies, Disease and Ancient Cultures,* Second Edition. Cambridge: Cambridge University Press; 237-262.

Frey S, Bongartz J, Giel D, Thelen A, and Hering P (2003) Ultrafast holographic technique for 3D in situ documentation of cultural heritage. *Proceedings of the SPIE International Society for Optical Engineering* 5146: 194-204.

Fricker EJ, Spigelman M, and Fricker CR (1997) The detection of Escherichia coli DNA in the ancient remains of Lindow Man using the polymerase chain reaction. *Letters in Applied Microbiology* 24: 351-354.

Gebühr M (1979) Das Kindergrab von Windeby -

Versuch einer "Rehabilitation". *Offa* 36:75-107.

Gebühr M (2002) *Moorleichen in Schleswig-Holstein.* Schleswig: Archäologisches Landesmuseum.

Gessel, P (2002) A 'despicable' affront to the dead. *Ottawa Citizen,* 12 December 2002.

Gill-Robinson HC (1996) Piglets in peat: experimental archaeology in the study of bog body preservation. In B Coles, J Coles, and M Schou Jørgensen (eds.): *Bog Bodies, Sacred Sites and Wetland Archaeology.* WARP Occasional Paper No. 12. Exeter: University of Exeter; 99-102.

Gill-Robinson HC (1998) Potential factors which allows the preservation of mammalian soft tissue in peat bogs. In T Malterer, K Johnson, and J Stewart (eds.): *Peatland Restoration and Reclamation: Techniques and Regulatory Considerations, Proceedings of the 1998 International Peat Symposium, Duluth, Minnesota.* Jyvasklya, Finland: International Peat Society; 185-188.

Gill-Robinson H.C (2000) *An Evaluation of Factors Contributing to the Preservation of Mammalian Soft Tissue in Peat Bogs.* Unpublished M.Phil Thesis, University of York, United Kingdom.

Gill-Robinson HC (2001) Peat and piglets: people and preservation. In A Millard (ed.): *Archaeological Sciences '97: Proceedings of the Conference held at the University of Durham, 2nd-4th September 1997.* British Archaeological Reports International Series 939 (BAR S939). Oxford: BAR Publishing; 160-163.

Gill-Robinson HC (2002) This little piggy went to Cumbria, this little piggy went to Wales: the tales of 12 piglets in peat. In J Mathieu (ed.): *Experimental Archaeology: Replicating Past Objects, Behaviors, and Processes.* British Archaeological Reports, International Series 1035 (BAR S1035). Oxford: BAR Publishing; 111-126.

Gill-Robinson HC (2003) Demographic data of bog bodies. In N Lynnerup, C Andreasen, and J Berglund (eds.): *Mummies in a New Millenium.* Copenhagen: Danish Polar Center; 43-46.

Gill-Robinson HC (In press) Bog bodies on display. In D Croes and BJ Coles (eds.): *Wet Sites Connections: Linking Indigenous Histories, Archaeology, and the Public.* Oxford: Oxbow Monographs.

Glob PV (1969) *The Bog People: Iron-Age Man Preserved.* London: Faber and Faber.

Grüner O (1979) Die "Moorleiche" von Windeby. *Offa* 36: 116-118.

Harck O (1973) Eisenzeitliche Muschelhaufen an der schleswigschen Ost- und Westküste. *Offa* 30: 40-50.

Healy F, and Housley RA (1992) Nancy was not alone: human skeletons of the Early Bronze Age from the Norfolk peat fen. *Antiquity* 66: 948-955.

Helmer R (1983) Die Moorleiche von Windeby. *Offa* 40: 345-362.

Holmes B (2001) Return of the mummy makers. *New Scientist* 172 (2320): 42-44.

Hunt J (1866) Observations on the influence of peat in destroying the human body, as shown by the discovery of human remains buried in peat in the Zetland. *The Anthropological Review* 4: 206-209.

Janaway RC, Wilson AS, Holland AD, and Baran EN (2003) Taphonomic changes to the buried body and associated materials in an upland peat environment: experiments using pig carcasses as human body analogues. In N Lynnerup, C Andreasen, and J Berglund (eds.): *Mummies in a New Millenium*. Copenhagen: Danish Polar Center; 56-59.

Ketelsen A (1966) Die Konservierung der Moorleiche von Datgen. *Der Preparator* 12:35-41.

Martin O (1967) Bericht uber die Untersuchung der Speisreste in der Moorleiche von Datgen. *Offa* 24: 77-78.

Mays S (1998) *The Archaeology of Human Bones*. London: Routledge.

Menon S (1997) The people of the bog. *Discover* 18(8): 60-67.

Micozzi MS (1991) *Postmortem Change in Human and Animal Remains: A Systematic Approach*. Springfield: Charles C Thomas.

Painter TJ (1991a) Preservation in peat. *Chemistry of Industry* 12: 451-424.

Painter, TJ (1991b) Lindow Man, Tollund Man and other peat bog bodies: The preservative and antimicrobial action of sphagnan, a reactive glycuronoglycan with carbohydrate polymers. *Carbohydrate Polymers* 15: 123-142.

Painter, TJ (1995) Chemical and microbiological aspects of the preservation process in sphagnum peat. In RC Turner and RG Scaife (eds): *Bog Bodies: New Discoveries and New Perspectives*. British Museum Press: London; 88-99.

Parker Pearson, M (1999) *The Archaeology of Death and Burial*. Phoenix Mill: Sutton Publishing.

Pieper, P (2003) Peat bog corpses. In A Bauerochse and H Haßmann (eds.): *Peatlands – Archaeological Sites – Archives of Nature – Nature Conservation – Wise Use. Proceedings of the Peatland Conference 2002 in Hannover, Germany*. Rahden, Westf: Verlag Marie Leidorf.; 107-114.

Saunders SR (2000) Subadult skeletons and growth-related studies. In MA Katzenberg and SR Saunders (eds.): *Biological Anthropology of the Human Skeleton*. New York: Wiley-Liss; 135-161.

Schiebler TH and Schaefer U (1961) Neue Moorleichenfunde in Schleswig-Holstein. *Die Umschau* 15: 466-467.

Schmidt, S (2002) Museum navigates ethical minefield in corpses exhibit. *National Post (Canada)*, 13 December 2002, A10.

Spigelman M, Fricker CR and Fricker EJ (1995) Addendum: Extracting DNA from Lindow Man's gut contents: modern technology looking for answers from ancient tissues. In RC Turner andRG Scaife (eds.): *Bog Bodies: New Discoveries and New Perspectives*. London: British Museum Press; 59-61.

Struve K (1967) Die Moorleiche von Datgen: Ein Diskussionsbeitrag zur Strafopferthese. *Offa* 24:33-76.

Sutter RC (2003) Nonmetric subadult skeletal sexing traits: I. A blind test of the accuracy of eight previously proposed methods prehistoric known-sex mummies from Northern Chile. *Journal of Forensic Science* 48(5): 927-935.

van der Plicht J, van der Sanden WAB, Aerts AT, and Streurman HJ (2004) Dating bog bodies by means of ^{14}C-AMS. *Journal of Archaeological Science* 31:471-491.

van der Sanden WAB (1993) Alfred Dieck und die niederländischen Moorleichen: einige kritische Randbemerkungen. *Die Kunde* N.F. 44: 127-139.

van der Sanden WAB (1996) *Through Nature to Eternity: The Bog Bodies of Northwest Europe*. Amsterdam: Batavian Lion International.

Von Haugwitz, K. *Die Moorleichen Schleswig-Holsteins: Dokumentation und Deutung, Unpublished Magister Thesis*, Universität Hamburg, Germany.

Wells C (1967) Pseudopathology. In D Brothwell and AT Sandison (eds.): *Diseases in Antiquity*. Springfield: Charles C Thomas; 5-19.

Beyond 'Man the Hunter': The Evidence from Windover (Florida, USA)

Beyond 'Man the Hunter'

Christine Hamlin

University of Wisconsin-Milwaukee, Department of Anthropology
Post Office Box 413, 290 Sabin Hall
Milwaukee, Wisconsin 53201
USA
chamlin@uwm.edu

Abstract

This paper examines the archaeological evidence for gender roles at the Windover site, Florida, USA. The recovery there of cultural materials not usually preserved in the archaeological record, in addition to a well-preserved and demographically complete skeletal population, provides a rare opportunity to study the division of labour by sex in an Archaic-period hunter-gatherer-fishing group. Artefacts from this mortuary pond site, one of only four such sites known in the world, include stone and bone weapons, textiles and the tools for their manufacture, wooden and turtle shell bowls, and the oldest *Lagenaria* species gourd recovered north of Mexico. Evidence from Windover suggests that rather than the 'man the hunter' model so entrenched in the public consciousness, this prehistoric population practiced patterns of task division which were much less rigidly differentiated, with tasks which have traditionally been considered strongly gendered, such as hunting and fishing, shared between the sexes.

Keywords: mortuary, gender, Archaic, hunter-gatherer, Florida, Windover

Introduction

The Windover archaeological site (8BR246) is a mortuary, or charnel, pond that was used between 8120±70 years BP and 6990±70 years BP (Doran & Dickel 1988a). Located approximately eight kilometres west of the Kennedy Space Centre, it is near Titusville on Florida's eastern coast (Fig. 1). This Early Archaic site has a number of distinctive features. It is one of only four known sites of its type in the world and is the earliest of these chronologically.[1] Because Windover was a wet-site, organic materials which do not typically survive in the archaeological record, wood, antler, textiles and bone, were well preserved. Indeed, one of the most extensive fibre arts collections in the Americas was recovered there (Doran & Dickel 1988b), as was one of the largest New World human skeletal populations dated to this period (Doran 1986). Together, the cultural and skeletal materials provide a rare opportunity to examine labour division in a prehistoric hunter-gatherer-fishing population. The resulting picture of life in this community suggests that models of task division at conventional prehistoric sites may be too rigid in their depiction of most activities as gendered. Many tasks, including those like hunting and fishing which have traditionally been considered strongly gendered, were

likely shared by the sexes at Windover. They may, then, have been shared at other prehistoric sites which do not exhibit the level of preservation found at Windover.

Given the rarity of this site type, a brief overview of site morphology and funerary behaviour at Windover is presented prior to a discussion of the artefact distribution patterning.

Site History and Morphology

The Windover site was discovered in 1982 during housing construction. Drs. Glen H. Doran and David N. Dickel (Department of Anthropology, Florida State University) co-directed site investigation, which was conducted through three field seasons (August through January of 1984, 1985 and 1986).

Windover is an isolated pond fed by subsurface groundwater and surface runoff (Doran & Dickel 1988b). The pond-bottom is peat, divided between four strata (Table 1). This peat deposit is unusual by virtue of both its depth and age. The majority of such deposits in central Florida began forming approximately 6,000 years ago and are 1.5 to 2 metres thick, while the Windover deposit dates from 10,750 years BP and is almost four metres in depth (Doran & Dickel 1988a). Approximately half of the Windover site was excavated and it is estimated that 100 to 150 burials survive in the remaining peat (Doran 1992: 127). The water and peat chemistry which combined to provide a preservation medium prior to excavation

---

[1] The other sites which exhibit mortuary evidence similar to that at Windover, Bay West (8CR200), Republic Groves Site (8HR4), and Little Salt Spring (8SO18), are all in Florida and all date to the Middle Archaic period (7,000-5,500 BP). For more information on these sites, see Clausen et al. 1979; Beriault et al. 1981; Wharton et al. 1981.

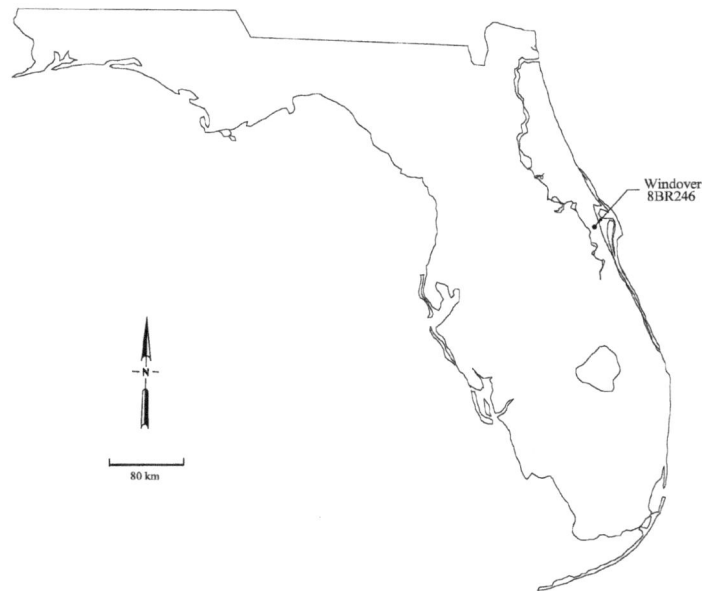

Figure 1.Location of the Windover Archaeological Site (8BR246), Florida, USA.
Image courtesy of Glen H. Doran and used with permission.

Table 1. Stratigraphy at the Windover Site, after Doran and Dickel (1988b: 367) and Doran (2002: 59-72).

Strata	Primary composition	Radiocarbon (^{14}C) dates (uncorrected)
Black peat	Sawgrass (*Cladium* species)	4,790±100 yrs BP (Beta-10763) to 6,070±90 yrs BP (Beta-13910)
Red-brown peat, upper substratum	*Cephalanthus, Myrica*, and *Salix* species	6,070±90 yrs BP (Beta-13910) to 7,050±80 yrs BP (Beta-14132)
Red-brown peat, lower substratum	*Cephalanthus, Myrica*, and *Salix* species	7,050±80 yrs BP (Beta-14132) to 7,550±90 yrs BP (Beta-19543)
Rubber peat	Freshwater snail shells (*P. duryi, P. scalaris*)	7,550±90 yrs BP (Beta-19543) to 8,770±90 yrs BP (Beta-19544)
Water-lily peat	Water-lily (*Nymphaea* species)	8,990±90 yrs BP (Beta-13908) to 10,750±190 yrs BP (Beta-13907)

(Flowers 1987) were re-established at the site and should ensure the continued survival of archaeologically significant materials.

Funerary Behaviour at Windover[2]

A great deal of information regarding the funerary rites of

those using the pond at Windover was preserved in its anaerobic matrix.

Table 2. Body Positioning at Windover.

Position	No. of Burials	%
Crouched burial	57	95
Extended burial	3	5
Total	60	100

Evidence suggests that the deceased were placed in the pond's peat bottom within 48 hours of death.[3] Burials

---

[2] The numbers presented in this section vary slightly from those presented at the September, 2003 conference. These changes result from a recent (July 2004) re-examination of the mortuary data by the author and Glen Doran. The gendered elements of mortuary behaviour at Windover will be discussed in detail in a forthcoming paper (Hamlin, in prep.).

[3] After 48 hours, brain structure begins to break down and decompositional gas vacuoles appear. 91 of the 169 individuals recovered at Windover had saponified brain tissue and nine had fully intact, though shrunken, brains. Analysis of this tissue utilising x-ray

were typically in crouched position, with 95% of individuals (n=60) in flexion (Table 2).[4]

Table 3. Body Positioning By Side at Windover.

Position	No. of Burials	%
Burial on left side	28	51.9
Burial on right side	18	33.3
Prone burial	8	14.8
Total	54	100

Of those for whom body placement information was available (n=54), half were interred on their left side, one-third on their right side, and the remainder were prone (Table 3).

Compass orientation for the body of the deceased[5] (n=66) varied, though placement of the head within an arc between southwest and west predominated (Table 4).

The recovery of textile matting or cloth with some of the deceased indicates that these individuals were wrapped in fabric – possibly shrouds or blankets – prior to being placed in the pond, while finer-gauged fabrics suggest that some individuals were buried clothed (Andrews et al. 1988). In a number of instances, wooden stakes which had been debarked, charred, and sharpened were recovered in association with burials (Doran & Dickel 1988a: 283). These may have served to mark individual graves or grave clusters (Newsom 1998), or to pin the deceased in place on the sloping pond bottom (Doran 1992). An inverted cone of unmodified wood was also sometimes erected over burials. Though the motivation for the placement of branches over the graves is unknown, the wood certainly functioned to deter scavengers (Dickel 1988: 7). Fewer than a dozen of the human bones recovered at Windover exhibited evidence of gnawing, though faunal remains indicate that several species of scavengers inhabited the pond during the period of its use for mortuary activities (Doran and Dickel 1988a: 273).

Table 4. Grave Orientation at Windover.

Head direction	No. of Burials	%
North	6	9.1
Northeast	2	3.0
East	6	9.1
Southeast	3	4.5
South	3	4.5
Southwest	16	24.2
West	27	40.9
Northwest	3	4.3
Total	66	100

The Windover pond appears to have been used for burial only during the late summer and/or early autumn (Doran 1992: 130). The analysis of stomach contents recovered at the site indicated that the types of plants and fruits ingested matured between July and October (Newsom 1998). Results of growth-ring analysis performed on wooden stakes from burials at the site were consistent with these findings (Newsom 1998). No evidence of Early Archaic habitation has been recovered in the areas adjacent to the pond (Doran & Dickel 1988b: 365), though this may well result from extensive construction work in the area prior to site discovery and during site survey and excavation.[6]

Submersion burial, as noted earlier, is exceedingly rare. The motivation for this unusual practice is unknown and no certain answer is forthcoming, as no cultural or genetic relationship has been demonstrated between those interred at Windover and any of the historic or modern Native American groups living in the south-eastern U. S. (Doran, pers. comm. 1999). Ethnographic studies of historic period Native Americans indicate that water was believed to act as a barrier to the souls of the deceased (Hall 1976), so perhaps interment in the pond at Windover was intended to keep the spirits of the dead from walking among the living. The well preserved cultural and skeletal materials at Windover can tell archaeologists much regarding the 'how' of mortuary behaviour there, but they remain mute on the 'why.'

Materials and Methodology

The remains of 169 individuals were recovered at Windover (Doran, pers. comm. 1995). This number includes 47 females, 48 males and 74 persons of undetermined sex (Table 5).

---

imaging, computerized axial tomography (CAT), and proton magnetic resonance imaging (MRI) showed that the recovered material retained its structural, cellular and molecular integrity (Doran et al. 1986; Hauswirth et al. 1991), and that gas vacuoles were not present (Dickel 1988: 2).

[4] 'In flexion' includes semi-flexed through tightly-flexed, using Ubelaker (1978) criteria. Disarticulation of the remaining burials at the site resulted from their migration downward along the uneven pond-bottom. The inflow of storm water into the pond and construction activities in the area prior to site discovery also likely played a role in burial disturbance (Dickel 1988: 2).

[5] Orientation was determined by the orientation of the vertebral spine "along a line determined by the superior point of contact of the pubic symphases of the pelvis, to the centre of the cranium (for flexed burials, as close as possible to the uppermost euryon" (Dickel 2002: 76-77).

---

[6] There is evidence of adjacent habitation at the Bay West (8CR200), Republic Groves (8HR4), and Little Salt Spring (8SO18) sites.

Table 5. Demographic Data for the Windover Population.

Age at Death	Total	Female	Male	Unknown
0-1	14			14
2-5	17			17
6-10	19			19
11-15	15			15
16-20	10	6	0	4
21-25	14	10	4	0
26-30	5	0	5	0
31-35	5	2	2	1
36-40	10	3	7	0
41-45	10	4	6	0
46 -50	15	7	8	0
51-55	3	2	1	0
56-60	7	2	4	1
61-65	10	3	7	0
66-70	2	2	0	0
71-75	1	0	1	0
Unknown	12	6	3	3
Total	169	47	48	74

Table 6. Demographic Profile of the Windover Sample Population

Age at Death	Total	Female	Male	Unknown
0-1	9			9
2-5	15			15
6-10	15			15
11-15	14			14
16-20	6	3	0	3
21-25	13	9	4	0
26-30	5	0	5	0
31-35	3	0	2	1
36-40	10	3	7	0
41-45	9	3	6	0
46-50	15	7	8	0
51-55	3	2	1	0
56-60	6	2	3	1
61-65	10	3	7	0
66-70	2	2	0	0
71-75	1	0	1	0
unknown	9	6	2	1
Total	145	40	46	59

Of the latter, 69 were subadults (age 17 or younger). Individuals ranged from neonatal/newborn to approximately 75 years in age (Table 5), and were present in numbers suggesting a balanced demographic representation. Sex and age in adults, and age in subadults, were assessed by Doran and Dickel (Doran, pers. comm. 2004) using standard nonmetric and metric features (cf., Steele & Bramblett 1988; White 1991) (Doran 2002: 36).[7]

This study includes 145 of the 169 individuals from the Wendover charnel pond (Table 6). The remaining 24 individuals were excluded because their remains were commingled, meaning that the remains of two or more individuals were recovered together and that any artefacts in association with this skeletal material could not be attributed with certainty to a given individual.[8]

Cultural materials were recovered in association with 82 of the 145 individuals. These included 23 females, 29 males, and 30 individuals of unknown sex (Table 7).

Table 7. Artefact Distribution by Sex and Age.

Age at Death	Total	Female	Male	Unknown
0-1	4			4
2-5	8			8
6-10	8			8
11-15	6			6
16-20	4	1	0	3
21-25	6	5	1	0
26-30	3	0	3	0
31-35	2	0	2	0
36-40	6	3	3	0
41-45	8	3	5	0
46 -50	12	6	6	0
51-55	2	1	1	0
56-60	4	1	2	1
61-65	5	1	4	0
66-70	2	2	0	0
71-75	1	0	1	0
Unknown	1	0	1	0
Total	82	23	29	30

---

[7] Age assessment for adults was based upon dental attrition rates (Walker 1978) correlated with pubic symphasis morphology and, when necessary, cranial suture closure (Buikstra and Ubelaker, 1994; Doran, 2002: 36). For subadults, age assessment was based upon radiographic assessment of dental development (Moorrees et al. 1963a, b) and epiphyseal union (Doran 2002: 36). All members of the population under age 17 were designated 'sex-unknown.
[8] Commingling is clearly, in most cases, the result of taphonomic processes (Dickel 1988: 2) [see endnote 3]. It is also possible that some of the commingled represent single-event burials of multiple individuals (Doran, pers. comm. 1998).

Chi-square (χ^2), (Voelker & Orton 1993: 128), was used to determine differences between the actual and expected artefact quantities for gendered distribution patterns. The sex of the deceased does not appear to have been a determinant of whether the individual was interred with grave goods, as there were no statistically significant differences in the frequency with which females and males were interred with grave goods ($\chi^2=0.27$, p>0.05).

Examination of the grave goods themselves proved a better indicator of gender ideology at Windover.

Rothschild (1990) and others have demonstrated that data regarding gender configurations can be recovered through analysis of the artefact assemblage using functional categorizations. The consistent association of a tool type with individuals of a particular gender likely indicates that members of said gender were responsible for a given task. Artefact types were determined by use-wear studies conducted on the Windover assemblage by Thomas Penders in 1997, and artefacts were assigned by the author to the following functional categories: domestic, fabricating and processing, hunting-related and weaponry, ornamental, unmodified materials, and other. A brief overview of each function category follows.

Domestic: Domestic artefacts are those items used in the execution of duties related to food preparation and textile manufacture (Table 8). Artefacts recovered at Windover that are included in this category: turtle shell containers, a wooden bowl, a wooden pestle, textiles of three types (cordage, fine-gauge woven fabric, matting), and a *Lagenaria* species gourd which had been modified for use as a container (Doran et al. 1990).

Fabricating and Processing: Artefacts in this category include all the tools necessary for the manufacture of the items required in daily life (Table 8). These include implements such as awls of various types, deer ulna butchering and burnishing tools, a faunal bone needle, antler pressure flakers and shark tooth drills. Also included are a number of the multipurpose pins/awls, a chert biface knife, and shark tooth gravers/scrapers.

Hunting-Related and Weaponry: Hunting-related artefacts and weaponry include atlatl components (cup/hooks, a dart shaft, weights), antler and lithic projectile points, and a snare trigger (Table 8). These items were primarily used in the procurement of seasonally available meat (Tuross et al. 1994), though they may also have been used against human opponents as possible evidence of interpersonal conflict was recovered at Windover (Dickel et al. 1989).

Ornamental: The only bodily adornments recovered *in situ* at the site were beaded necklaces (Table 8), and these were quite rare. Beads were manufactured from four materials, antler, fish vertebrae, shell, and Sabal Palmetto seeds.

Unmodified Material: This category includes unmodified faunal bone and shell (Table 8). These inclusions may represent food offerings placed with the deceased for use during their journey to the realm of the dead or in their afterlife, or may have been provided for use in the manufacture of tools or ornaments in the afterlife.

Other: The ubiquitous 'other' category encompasses all items not assigned to the artefact categories discussed above (Table 8). Bird bone tubes, which may have been used for smoking tobacco and medicinal herbs or as beads for bodily ornamentation (Penders 1997: 121-122), were present, as were butchered faunal bones, which were likely food inclusions which then could have been used by the deceased for the manufacture of tools in the afterlife. Miscellaneous modified antler and modified deer metapodials recovered in association with burials at

Table 8. Artefact Types by Function Category.

Domestic	Fabricating and processing	Hunting-related and weaponry	Ornamental	Unmodified materials	Other
turtle shell containers	awls of various type	atlatl components (cup/hook, dart shaft, weight)	beads: shell	unmodified shell	bird bone tubes
wooden bowl	deer ulna butchering and burnishing tools	antler tine projectile points	beads: antler	unmodified faunal bone	butchered faunal bones
wooden pestle	faunal bone needle	lithic projectile points	beads: fish vertebrae		modified antler and deer metapodials
textile: cordage	antler pressure flakers	snare trigger	beads: Sabal Palmetto seed		botanical remains (seed cache, Opuntia pad)
textile: fine-gauge woven fabric	shark tooth drills				wooden stakes
textile: matting	multipurpose pin/awls				
gourd container	chert biface knife				
	shark tooth graver/scrapers				

Windover may also have been intended for tool production in the afterlife, as both antler and metapodials were materials from which tools were manufactured. Seed caches were, in some instances, clearly the remnants of food placed with the deceased, while others may represent stomach contents. An intact *Opuntia* species (prickly pear) pad was a probable food offering, as seeds from this fruit were common in stomach contents recovered at Windover (Doran & Dickel 1988b: 368). Lastly, the 'other' category includes the wooden stakes used to pin or mark the wet-site burials.

Results and Discussion

Statistically significant differences in artefact distribution patterns for females and males were noted when the Windover assemblage was analysed using functional categorizations. The disproportionate distribution of

artefacts designated 'hunting-related and weaponry' (χ^2=6.63, p<0.01) and 'fabricating and processing' (χ^2=6.63, p<0.01) in favour of males suggests that males may have been primarily responsible for these duties. These findings, however, provide only the broadest indication of daily task division at Windover. A more nuanced picture is possible when one examines the distribution of artefacts by type. While small sample size precluded the application of statistical techniques to artefact type distribution patterning, the findings presented below suggest possible trends and may serve as patterns against which to test other mortuary samples when they become available.

Antler-tine projectile points from the 'hunting-related and weaponry' category were recovered in association with both sexes. Only females, however, were recovered with barbed antler projectile points and only males were found with lithic projectile points (Table 9). Atlatl components were also recovered only in association with males (Table 9). Penders (1997: 155) has suggested that antler points may have been used in the procurement of small mammals, reptiles and fish, while implements such as lithic points and atlatls were likely used for hunting large terrestrial game such as deer and marine mammals such as manatee. Both sexes, then, may have hunted small game and speared fish, while males may have been primarily responsible for hunting larger game.

The attribution of task by tool analysis is more difficult for items designated 'fabricating and processing.' That several artefact types from this function category were used by both sexes is certain, deer ulna gouge/butchering tools, antler pressure flakers, bevelled-tipped burnisher/awls, modified deer metapodials, and a number of other implement types were recovered in association with both males and females. Use-wear studies, though, indicate that many tools were multi-purpose implements, and whether the tools were used by both sexes for the same task is not known. The materials upon which the

tools were used may also have varied depending upon the tool-user's gender. Artefacts manufactured from stone were recovered only in association with males at Windover and those manufactured from shell only with females. Penders (1997: 117) posited that antler pressure flakers could have been used on both of these materials. The gender of the tool-user may, then, have determined the material upon which a tool was used or the task to which it was put.

Table 9. Single-Gender Artefact Types.

Types with males	Types with females
lithic projectile point	barbed antler projectile point
atlatl components	turtle-shell container
hollow-point awl	butchered faunal bone
antler perforator/punch	textile bag/container
bone needle	*Opuntia* pad
deer ulna gouge/burnishing tool	bird-bone tube
mammal canine graver/burnisher	shell necklace bead
shark-tooth drill	shark-tooth graver/scraper
misc. modified antler	

A number of artefact types in the fabricating and processing category were gendered by exclusive association with a single sex. Hollow-point awls, for instance, were found only in association with males at Windover (Table 9). These were likely used in the manufacture of fishing nets and lines (Penders, 1997: 134), suggesting that males may have manufactured the nets and lines used by both genders, or possibly that males were responsible for catching fish in these ways.

That food preparation may have been as task gendered female is supported by the exclusive association of females and subadults with turtle shell containers, which Penders (1997) indicated may have served as mortars, and with butchered faunal bone (Table 9). Use-wear also suggests the use of turtle shells as rigid containers, an item useful in gathering vegetative foodstuffs. Two globular textile bags were recovered at Windover, one in association with a female and the other with an unsexed subadult, while the sole *Opuntia* species pad recovered at the site was with a female (Table 9). *Opuntia* seeds were, as noted earlier, a common constituent of the seed caches thought to be food offerings and stomach contents. While a single bag, one *Opuntia* pad, and the possible use of turtle-shells as rigid containers cannot be used to assert that females were the sole gatherers of plant materials for the Windover community, it certainly suggests that they were performing this task. That females participated in the procurement of plant material at Windover is further strengthened by the exclusive association of females with bird bone tubes, which may have served as smoking tubes for medicinal herbs (Penders 1997: 163) or for ritual use in the removal of bodily or spiritual contaminants (Lewis & Lewis, 1984; Hudson & Blackburn 1986). The mortars used in food preparation could also have been used to prepare plant medicines for administration through the bird bone tubes (Penders 1997: 163). The mortar, textile bag, and bird bone tube may, then, have functioned in a mortuary context as symbols of the shamanic or healing role served by certain women in the community.

Conclusion

The analysis of the Windover artefact assemblage by functional category provides general information about task division in this community. The larger proportional representation of artefacts designated 'hunting-related and weaponry' suggests that males may have been primarily responsible for the procurement of non-vegetative foodstuffs (meat and fish), while the larger number of male burials with 'fabricating and processing' tools likely indicates that males may have been responsible for the processing of faunal materials for the fabrication of tools. Though the artefacts associated with these tasks are more common with males, however, they were not exclusive to them. Artefacts recovered from female burials suggest that females hunted small mammals, speared fish and reptiles, and collected plant material for preparation as foodstuffs and medicines, while males hunted small and large mammals and procured fish by spear and net. The exclusive presence of stone implements with males may indicate that they alone were responsible for the collection of the raw material for and manufacture of these items. Similarly, the exclusive presence of shell ornaments with females may indicate that they were solely responsible for the collection of shellfish (or simply that ornaments manufactured from shell were gendered female). The recovery of butchering and filleting tools with both sexes suggests these were non-gendered tasks, though the presence of gendered projectile point types raises the possibility that each gender may have butchered only the species they procured. The association of tools related to textile manufacture with both sexes suggests that this too was a non-gendered task, though the type of textile produced may have differed by sex, with males producing fishing nets while females made some of the other types of textiles recovered at Windover.

The analysis of artefacts by function and type suggests that the division of labour at Windover does not fit the 'Man the Hunter' model so entrenched in the public consciousness, in that males were not likely the only hunters. Instead, it appears that tasks were not as strongly gender-coded as were the tools used to perform the task and the association of a particular artefact or material type with a given gender. The mental picture of males as the primary purveyors of protein is further undermined by

the results of carbon and nitrogen bone-collagen levels from human skeletal material recovered at Windover, which indicate that this population was heavily reliant on riverine protein resources, with aquatic birds (duck, osprey, blue heron), turtles, and catfish the probable primary protein sources, and secondary reliance on the small mammals that exploit this environment, such as raccoons and opossums (Tuross et al.1994: 295). The recovery of tools appropriate for the procurement of small mammals and fish with both sexes suggests that both were indeed contributing hunted and fished resources to the community. No significant dietary reliance on either large or small terrestrial game, such as deer or rabbit, was demonstrated through bone-collagen analysis (Tuross et al. 1994: 295), though the presence of deer bone and antler tools certainly indicates that deer were a valued resource for this population. The bone/antler/dentary assemblage and the results of archaeobotanical and bone-collagen analyses together show the Windover population to be a resourceful hunting-gathering-fishing population in which both genders shared the tasks necessary to effectively exploit a rich resource base.

Acknowledgements

The author wishes to thank Glen Doran, for material and unpublished data on the Windover site, and Rebecca Redfern, for presenting this paper at the conference in the author's absence.

Literature Cited

Andrews RL, Adovasio JM, and Harding DG (1988) *An Interim Report in the Conservation and Analysis of Perishables from the Windover Archaeological Project, Florida.* Paper submitted to the Windover Archaeological Project, Florida State University, Tallahassee, FL.

Beriault J, Carr R, Stipp J, Johnson R, and Meeder J (1981) The Archaeological Salvage of the Bay West Site, Collier County, Florida. *Florida Anthropology* 34(2): 39-58.

Buikstra JE, and Ubelaker DH (eds) (1994) *Standards for Data Collection from Human Skeletal Remains.* Fayetteville: Arkansas Archaeological Research Series, No. 44. Arkansas Archaeological Survey

Clausen CJ, Cohen AD, Emiliani C, Holman JA, and Stipp JJ (1979) Little Salt Spring, Florida: A Unique Underwater Site. *Science* 203: 609-613.

Dickel DN (1988) *Analysis of Mortuary Patterns at the Windover Site.* Paper submitted to the Windover Archaeological Research Project, Florida State University, Tallahassee, FL.

Dickel DN (2002) Analysis of Mortuary Patterns. In *Windover: Multidisciplinary Investigations of an Early Archaic Florida Cemetery*, Doran, G (ed.). Gainesville, FL: University of Florida Press; 73-96.

Dickel DN, Aker CG, Barton BK, and Doran GH (1989) An Orbital Floor and Ulna Fracture from the Early Archaic of Florida. *Journal of Paleopathology* 2(3): 165-170.

Doran GH (1986) *National Register of Historic Places Inventory – Nomination Form*. On file with the Florida Department of State, Tallahassee, FL.

Doran GH (1992) Problems and Potential of Wet Sites in North America: The Example of Windover. In B Coles (ed.): *The Wetland Revolution in Prehistory*. Exeter, England: University of Exeter; 125-134.

Doran GH (ed). (2002) The Windover Radiocarbon Chronology. In *Windover: Multidisciplinary Investigations of an Early Archaic Florida Cemetery*, Doran, G (ed.). Gainesville, FL: University of Florida Press; 59-72.

Doran GH and Dickel DN (1988a) Radiometric Chronology of the Archaic Windover Archaeological Site (8BR246). *The Florida Anthropologist* 41(3): 365-380.

Doran GH, and Dickel DN (1988b) Multidisciplinary Investigations at the Windover Site. In BA Purdy (ed): *Wet Site Archaeology*. Caldwell, NJ: Telford Press; 263-289.

Doran GH, Dickel DN, Ballinger W Jr., Agee OF, Laipis PJ, and Hauswirth WW (1986) Anatomical, Cellular, and Molecular Analysis of 8000-Year-Old Human Brain Tissue from the Windover Archaeological Site. *Nature* 323(6091): 803-806.

Doran GH, Dickel DN, and Newsom LA (1990) A 7,290-Year-Old Bottle Gourd from the Windover Site, Florida. *American Antiquity* 55(2): 354-360.

Flowers J (1987) *Water Analysis of Samples from the Windover Pond*. Report submitted to Windover Archaeological Research Project, Florida State University, Tallahassee, FL.

Hall RL (1976) Ghosts, Water Barriers, Corn, and Sacred Enclosures in the Eastern Woodlands. *American Antiquity* 41(3): 360-364.

Hauswirth WW, Dickel CN, Doran GH, Laipis PJ, and Dickel DN (1991) 8000-Year-Old Brain Tissue from the Windover Site: Anatomical, Cellular, and Molecular Analysis. In DJ Ortner and AC Aufderheide (eds.): *Human Paleopathology: Current Syntheses and Future Options*. Washington, DC: Smithsonian Institution Press; 60-72.

Hudson T, and Blackburn TC (1986) *The Material Culture of the Chumash Interaction Sphere, Volume 4: Ceremonial Paraphernalia, Games, and Amusement*. Santa Barbara, CA: Ballena Press.

Lewis TMN, and Lewis M Kneberg (1984) *Hiwassee Island: An Archaeological Account of Four Tennessee Indian Peoples*. 5th edition. Knoxville, TN: University of Tennessee Press.

Moorrees CFA, Fanning EA, and Hunt EE Jr. (1963a) Age Variation of Formation Stages of Ten Permanent Teeth. *Journal of Dental Research* 42: 1490-1502.

Moorrees CFA, Fanning EA, and Hunt EE Jr. (1963b) Formation and Resorption of Three Deciduous Teeth in Children. *American Journal of Physical Anthropology* 21: 205-213.

Newsom LA (1998) *The Paleoethnobotany of Windover (8BR246): An Archaic Period Mortuary Site in Central Florida*. Paper submitted to the Windover Archaeological Project, Florida State University, Tallahassee, FL.

Penders TE (1997) *A Study of the Form and Function of the Bone and Antler Artifacts from the Windover Archaeological Site (8BR246), Brevard County, Florida*. Master's thesis, Florida State University, Department of Anthropology, Tallahassee, FL.

Rothschild NA (1990) *Prehistoric Dimensions of Status: Gender and Age in Eastern North America*. NY, NY: Garland Publishing Co.

Steele DG, and Bramblett CA (1988) *The Anatomy and Biology of the Human Skeleton*. College Station, TX: Texas A&M University Press.

Tuross N, Fogel ML, Newsom LA, and Doran GH (1994) Subsistence in the Florida Archaic: The Stable-Isotope and Archaeobotanical Evidence from the Windover Site. *American Antiquity* 59(2): 288-303.

Ubelacker DH (1978) *Human Skeletal Remains: Excavation, Analysis,* Interpretation. Chicago, IL: Aldine.

Voelker DH and Orton PZ (1993) *Statistics*. Lincoln, NB: Cliffs Notes, Inc.

Walker P (1978) Quantitative Analysis of Dental Attrition Rates in the Santa Barbara Channel Area. *American Journal of Physical Anthropology* 48: 101-106.

Wharton BR, Ballo GR, and Hope ME (1981) The Republic Groves Site, Hardee County, Florida. *Florida Anthropologist* 34(2): 59-80.

White TD (1991) *Human Osteology*. San Diego, CA: Academic Press.

Changing Views About The Local Evolution Of Human Populations In The Southeastern Pampas Of Argentina During The Holocene

Human Evolution in the Argentine Pampas

G. Barrientos[1], S. Perez[2], V. Bernal[3], P. González[3], M. Béguelin[2], M. Del Papa[3]

[1] CONICET, Instituto Nacional de Antropología y Pensamiento Latinoamericano; Facultad de Ciencias Naturales y Museo, Universidad Nacional de La Plata, República Argentina.
[2] CONICET, Facultad de Ciencias Naturales y Museo, Universidad Nacional de La Plata, República Argentina.
[3] Facultad de Ciencias Naturales y Museo, Universidad Nacional de La Plata, República Argentina.

barrient@museo.fcnym.unlp.edu.ar

Abstract: The archaeological models and hypotheses derived to explain the local evolution of hunter-gatherer populations in the southeastern Pampas of Argentina (formulated in the last 20 years) assumed that it was a rather continuous and transformative process. To a large extent, this view can be considered as an enduring legacy of early processual archaeology, in which biocultural evolution was mainly envisioned as a process of internal, adaptive adjustment. Based on recent developments in metapopulation biology and evolutionary geography, and with analysis of archaeological and bioarchaeological evidence, we propose an alternative view. According to this, the aboriginal population history of the Pampas was not a continuous process that somehow started in the Late Pleistocene and finished in recent times, but a punctuated one, in which depopulation, colonisation and population replacement events may have occurred more than once during the last 13,000 years. In this paper we present and discuss the evidence — at both regional and supra-regional scale — supporting this claim (e.g., temporal distribution of calibrated ^{14}C-ages and human craniofacial morphology), exploring their implications for the archaeological study of the human peopling of the Pampas.

Key words: Holocene, Pampas, hunter-gatherers, population dynamics, metapopulations, radiocarbon calibration, human morphology.

Introduction

During the last twenty years, the prevailing view about the local evolution of hunter-gatherer populations in the southeastern Pampas of Argentina (37°-39° South Lat., 57°-63° West Long.) was one in which such a process was envisioned as continuous, transformative and, to some extent, adaptive (Martínez, 1999, 2002; Politis, 1984; Politis and Madrid, 2001). However, recent theoretical developments in metapopulation biology (Hanski, 1999; Hanski and Gilpin, 1997) and evolutionary geography (Lahr and Foley, 1998) challenge that view. According to these conceptual advances, local population history is almost never the result of a gradual, continuous process.[1] Human populations, like any other

biological populations, are subjected to largely stochastic events (Lande, 1993; Lande, et al. 1998; Liebhold and Bascompte, 2003). These alternatively lead to the expansion or contraction, growth or decline, diversification or homogenisation, isolation or integration, persistence or extinction (see Fix, 1999). The interrelationship between and within these developments shapes the tempo and mode of genetic and cultural change. Our main argument here is that the aboriginal population history of the Pampas, particularly of its southeastern portion, was not a continuous, gradual process that somehow started in the Late Pleistocene and finished in recent, historical times. Instead, we consider it as a rather punctuated one in which depopulation, colonisation and population replacement events may have occurred more than once during the last 13,000 years. The evidence supporting this claim is related to: a) the temporal distribution of calibrated ^{14}C ages, and b) the morphological differences between diachronic human skeletal samples. The aim of this paper is to present both lines of evidence, discussing their implications for the archaeological study of the human peopling of the

---

[1] Ames (2000) distinguished two levels at which continuities or discontinuities can be recognised: a) cultural traditions, and b) chains of evidence. At the first level, cultural continuities means that cultural transmission of a particular suite of cultural traits from one generation to another was continuous. A discontinuity means that one cultural system ceased to be transmitted, and was replaced for whatever reason by another. At the second level, the presence of gaps or breaks in the chain of evidence (such as lengthy gaps between radiocarbon dates, occupational hiatus at the local or regional scale, etc.), may be clues to discontinuities in the historical or evolutionary connection between

---

ancestral and descent cultures or populations. The focus in this paper is on the latter level of analysis.

Pampas. In order to put such a discussion into context we first present a brief account of the historical trends in the archaeology and bioanthropology of the southeastern Pampas, and an outline of the conceptual background to the archaeological study of past human populations and metapopulations.

Historical Trends in the Archaeological and Bioanthropological Study of the Human Peopling of the Pampas

Archaeological and bioanthropological research in the Argentine Pampas began with the pioneering work of F. Moreno, E. Zeballos and F. Ameghino in the 1870s (Politis, 1988a, 1995). It was only in the last five decades, however, that the main bulk of the currently available archaeological database was collected and integrated into interpretative and explicative models regarding the evolution of the aboriginal hunter-gatherer societies during the Late Pleistocene and the Holocene. As early as the 1930s, but particularly after World War II, the culture area approach promoted by the German-Austrian diffusionist school or *Kulturkreislehre* (Barnard, 2000; Willey and Sabloff, 1980) dominated archaeology and anthropology in the region (Politis, 1995). In the Pampas, as in many other regions of Argentina, the historic, antimaterialistic and antievolutionary view adopted by the early adherents of this school and their disciples (Boschín and Llamazares, 1984; Carnese et al., 1991/1992), imposed an interpretative and explanatory model in which diffusion and migration were the main mechanisms accounting for cultural and biological change (e.g., Bórmida, n.d.; Imbelloni, 1938; Menghin and Bórmida, 1950; Sanguinetti de Bórmida, 1970). Morphological types, conceived as discovered (i.e., natural) rather than methodologically imposed groupings of biological forms, and representing fixed and harmonious genotypic assemblages (Bórmida, 1953/1954: 82), were proposed as the major units for biological description and comparison (Bórmida, 1953-1954; Imbelloni, 1938).

The influence of New Archaeology or the processual approach arrived late to Argentina, in part as a consequence of the enduring prestige of the *Kulturkreislehre* in most of the country's academic circles (Politis, 1988a, 1995). It was only in the late 1970s that a new generation of archaeologists began to systematically incorporate concepts and models developed by American archaeology. As a reaction to the diffusionist and ecumenical point of view of the *Kulturkreislehre* (Willey and Sabloff, 1980: 107-108), an overall, albeit implicit, rejection of diffusion and migration occurred. In the Pampas, local transformation *via* cultural adaptation was the main mechanism of cultural change proposed (Martínez, 1999; Politis, 1984, 1985). Biological disruption and discontinuity were considered as rather unimportant sources of archaeological variation, and cultural evolution was mainly viewed as a process of internal (i.e., organisational) adjustment through which culture systems adapted themselves to their environment and changes in that environment (Martínez, 1999, 2002; Politis, 1985, 1988b). In very few instances (Martínez, 1999; Politis, 1984; Politis and Madrid, 2001), were explicit references to the populational dynamics responsible for or responsive to those transformational changes (e.g., demographic fluctuations) made.

It is significant that the models of the peopling of the Pampas with the greatest influence, despite their paradigmatic differences (e.g., Bórmida, n.d.; Menghin, 1963; Menghin and Bórmida, 1950; Politis, 1984), highlighted many similar traits shared by different, diachronic archaeological contexts, indeed proposing the existence of cultural traditions[2] to account for those similarities. From the perspective of the *Kulturkreislehre*, and based mainly upon technological criteria, Menghin and Bórmida (Bórmida, n.d.; Menghin, 1963; Menghin and Bórmida, 1950), advanced the hypothesis of a cultural tradition of "inferior hunters" in the Pampas (called the *Tandiliense*). Influenced by the American school, and covering a significant part of the southeastern Pampas, Politis (1984; see discussion in Politis and Madrid, 2001: 743-746) proposed the existence of a cultural tradition termed the *Interserrana*. This model was formulated on the basis of several technological and economic traits shared by diachronic archaeological components defined at different sites (Politis, 1984, 1988b). The traits included the dominance of quartzite as a raw material, the use of flakes as blanks, with subsequent unifacial reduction, the exploitation of *Lama guanicoe* (guanaco) as principal prey, and mammals such as *Ozotoceros bezoarticus* (small deer), *Lagostomus maximus* (large rodent), species of armadillos, and the bird *Rhea americana* (greater rhea) as secondary prey (Politis, 1984: 296-303). The notion of tradition, constructed on the basis of similarities shared by diachronic archaeological contexts, strongly contributed to the imposition of a concept of continuity in the human peopling of the Pampas. The perceived temporal differences in the archaeological record, as organised into industries (Bórmida, n.d.) or phases (Politis, 1984, 1988b; Silveira, 1992), were mainly conceived as representing local transformations due to different causes (e.g., environmental change, diffusion, cultural adaptation), and not as a probable reflection of major populational or social disruptions.

---

[2] The term tradition has been defined by Willey and Phillips (1958: 38) as "a [primarily] temporal continuity represented by persistent configurations in single technologies or other systems of related forms", constituting a useful tool in archaeological research into cultural stability. Traditions demonstrated "the staying power of certain regional-cultural ideas" (Willey, 1945: 55), thus reflecting the transmission or diffusion of such ideas across time (Lyman et al., 1997: 193).

Table 1. Principal differences between recent approaches to the archaeology of the southeastern Pampas of Argentina.

	Early 1980s to late 1990s	Present
Spatial scale	local, regional	regional, supra-regional
Population units	implicit, non defined	explicitly defined
Nature of the peopling	Continuous, gradual	discontinuous
Cultural change	transformation, adaptation	variation, competition, replacement
Evidence	archaeological	archaeological, bioarchaeological

Since the middle 1990s, side by side with other theoretical perspectives (see Politis and Madrid, 2001), explicit evolutionary approaches have begun to be applied to the interpretation of the Pampean archaeological and bioarchaeological records. As a consequence, a renewed interest in defining biological units at the population level arose in order to understand the pattern of variation in the archaeological record. The explicit application of principles from human behavioural ecology (Cronk et al., 2000; Smith and Winterhalder, 1992), dual inheritance theory (Boyd and Richerson, 1985; Cavalli-Sforza and Feldman, 1981) and evolutionary geography (Lahr, 2002; Lahr and Foley, 1998) has led to the consideration of population history and dynamics as a major source of archaeological variation (Barrientos, 1997, 2001, 2002; Barrientos and Perez, 2002, 2004a, 2004b; Martínez, 2002; Martínez and Mackie, 2003). Table 1 summarises the principal differences characterising the field at the level of the patial scale of analysis, the population units addressed, the concepts about the nature of the peopling, the mechanisms of cultural change involved, and the nature of the evidence used in order to test the specific archaeological hypotheses.

The Archaeological Study of Prehistoric Human Populations and Metapopulations

In previous papers, Barrientos and Perez (2002, 2004a) proposed that the hunter-gatherers groups that inhabited the southeastern Pampas during the Holocene were members of local populations belonging to geographically extended metapopulations. A metapopulation can be defined as a group of local populations characterised by relatively asynchronous and independent dynamics, resulting from their geographic separation, but ultimately linked to each other by the migration of individuals (Levins, 1969; cf. Hanski, 1999). In a bioarchaeological approach, the empirical referents used for the recognition of prehistoric human populations or metapopulations are skeletal remains corresponding to individuals that exhibit variable degrees of preservation and integrity. Such referents are the results of depositional events occurring at particular sites or regions and at different rates, across a time lapse that frequently comprises a number of generations and different or variable demographic regimes (i.e., they are affected by the so called "lineage effect"; Cadien et al., 1976).

Indeed, the samples of past human populations are allochronic units conformed by individuals belonging to evolving lineages whose temporal and spatial boundaries are, more often than not, diffuse.

From a bioarchaeological standpoint it is highly probable that we obtain scattered skeletal samples, especially in the context of hunter-gatherer populations. Then, it becomes necessary to assess — using different lines of evidence (e.g., zooarchaeological, technological, isotopic) — the geographic superposition of the potential ranges (the latter defined at different spatial and temporal scales, e.g., annual ranges, life-cycle territories, etc.) of the represented individuals. This implies that is desirable to define a localised population sample (LPS) (Sokal and Crovello, 1992: 38) in terms of the pattern and degree of mobility inferred for each population or set of populations under investigation. Clearly, a localised population is not a local population in the conventional biological sense (i.e. that used in population genetics) as all that is required to define it is a spatial, temporal or ecological connection between individuals, and not a genetic connection derived from reproductive relationships. The biological meaning of a sample drawn from a localised population is one of a probabilistic nature, whose probability level is conferred by some criterion of phenetic similarity (e.g., homogeneity; Sokal and Crovello, 1992: 39). The degree of similarity between and within different LPSs can be measured using multivariate statistical techniques applied to the analysis of continuous and discontinuous morphological traits (e.g., discriminant analysis; Pietrusewsky, 2000; van Vark and Schaasfma, 1992). Diverse LPSs can present a different degree of phenetic similarity at different spatial and temporal scales. From a spatial point of view, it is possible to conceive of the existence of a metapopulation sample (MPS) at a regional or supra-regional scale of analysis. A MPS is composed by a set of contemporaneous LPSs, geographically separated one each other and, ideally, with a degree of mean phenetic differentiation between-LPSs less than the within-LPSs mean phenetic differentiation. From a temporal standpoint, successive LPSs or MPSs can present a distinct degree of phenetic similarity according to the populational dynamics occurring at each geographic setting (e.g., populational continuity, local extinction, recolonisation by members of the same or different metapopulation, etc.). As a general expectation, we can

Table 2. Geographic provenience, geologic age and size of the fourteen samples of human crania analysed.

Region	N	Sample	Age (ka CAL BP)	n
SE Pampas	1	SE Pampa EMH (Early/Middle Holocene)	9-7	5
	2	SE Pampa ELH (Early Late Holocene)	3.2-1.9	6
	3	SE Pampa LLH (Late Late Holocene)	0.9-0.5	6
NE Pampas	4	Parana Delta	1-0.5?	9
NE Patagonia	5	San Blas	1.3-0.5	10
	6	Isla Gama	1.3-0.5	6
	7	Rio Negro PL (tabular erect deformation)	1.3-0.5	24
	8	Rio Negro TO (tabular oblique deformation)	3-1.5?	7
	9	Rio Negro C (circular deformation)	>3?	14
	10	Rio Negro UD (un-deformed)	?	19
	11	Chubut PL (tabular erect deformation)	1.3-0.5	38
	12	Chubut UD (un-deformed)	?	23
SW Patagonia	13	NW Santa Cruz	1.1-0.3	5
Southern Cuyo	14	Mendoza UD (un-deformed)	2	28
	15	Mendoza PL (tabular erect deformation)	1-0.5	9
Northern Cuyo	16	San Juan	?	12
Northwest	17	Catamarca	1-0.5	10
Total				231

say that in the case of continuity at the regional (populational) or supra-regional (metapopulational) level, significant phenetic differences between successive LPSs or MPSs should not exist. Similarly, when processes such as local extinction followed by recolonisation by members of the same metapopulation, or the geographic expansion of a local population over the spatial range of another local population of the same metapopulation, significant phenetic differences between successive MPSs should not exist either. Conversely, when local extinctions or geographic contractions were followed by recolonisation by members of a different metapopulation, the probability of detecting significant phenetic differences will consequently increase.

As it is likely that the Pampas had significant ecological or physical barriers promoting population isolation, gene flow due to migration from and to neighbouring areas may have been an effective mechanism enabling the formation of metapopulations at the supra-regional level. The hypothesised geographic range of such metapopulations includes the north of Patagonia, the Dry Pampas, southern Cuyo, the northeastern Pampas and, probably, Sierras Centrales (Barrientos and Perez, 2002) (Fig. 1). These metapopulations may have been sensitive to the selective conditions imposed by the environmental (e.g., climatic, faunal, vegetational, etc.) and ecological (e.g., habitat reduction or extension, competition, etc.) variations that occurred during the Holocene. In response, they may have changed by means of demographic regulation resulting in their contraction or expansion and, eventually, in their local extinction and replacement, thus affecting the continuity of biological and cultural processes at the regional scale. From the theoretical

perspective of evolutionary geography (Lahr and Foley, 1998), the evolution of diversity within any one lineage is shaped by both expansion/dispersal and contraction/extinction processes. In particular, one of the most important determinants for the evolution of dispersal rates is the extinction risk to which local populations are exposed (Lahr, 2002). They result in empty or thinly populated patches, the existence of which makes dispersal both feasible and profitable. For these reasons, increasing extinction risks at the regional level are expected to select for higher dispersal rates at the metapopulational (i.e. supra-regional) level (Parvinen et al., 2003).

Materials and Methods

Radiocarbon data
The radiocarbon datasets available for any given region can be used, if properly treated and discussed, to assess demographic processes through time (e.g., Ames, 2000; Bocquet-Appel and Demars, 2000; Gamble et al. 2003; Housley et al., 1997, 2000; Pettitt, 2000; Pettitt and Pike, 2001; Rick, 1987). The changing frequencies of radiocarbon dates can be interpreted as proxy measures of the intensity of past human activity at the regional level. More importantly, significant solutions of continuity in a series of radiocarbon dates can constitute valuable clues of population disruption events if sampling biases can be confidently discarded (Barrientos, 1997; Barrientos and Perez, 2004a). In a previous paper (Barrientos and Perez, 2004a) we presented the criteria used to screen the full radiocarbon dataset then available for the southeastern Pampas (n= 107; Politis and Madrid, 2001) in order to obtain a useful and reliable sample to perform statistical

analyses aimed at detecting significant gaps in the series of uncalibrated dates. On the resulting series of 72 dates, two major significant gaps were detected: the first between 8620 and 8060 ^{14}C years BP, and the second between 5960 and 5060 ^{14}C years BP (Barrientos and Perez, 2004a). In the present study we proceeded to add to that series six recently published dates that fulfilling the standardised criteria described in Barrientos and Perez (2004a), and to calibrate the resulting 78 determinations using the CALPAL_A package (Weninger et al., 2003). This software allows the showing of calibrated ^{14}C-ages in a graphical context with some specific, purposely selected paleoclimate proxies. The advantage of this basically graphical-explorative approach is that events and processes can be studied in comparison with changes in climate and environment (Weninger et al., 2003). The calibrated results were represented in a 2-d dispersion calibration graph showing the probability distribution of the ^{14}C-ages on the calendar time scale (i.e., calibrated age distribution) (Weninger, 1997). As a paleoclimate proxy of hemispheric significance (cf. Masson et al., 2000), we used the Lake Vostok ice-core temperature curve (east Antarctica; 78°28' South Lat., 106°48' East Long.), covering the period 0-400 ka CAL BP (Petit et al., 1999).

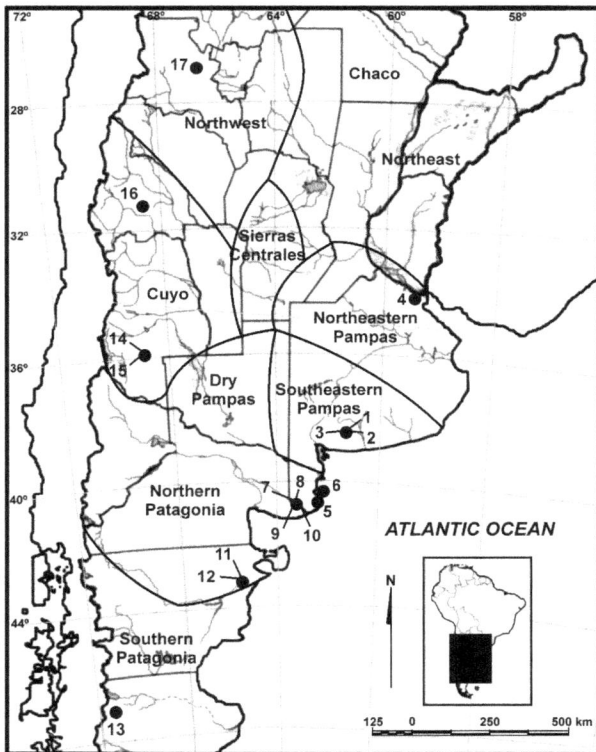

Figure 1. Map showing the distribution of the regions and samples of human skeletal remains discussed in the text. The numbers correspond to the sample numbers in Table 2.

Morphological data

In order to assess the degree of morphological affinity between the diachronic skeletal series from the southeastern Pampas, three LPSs composed of adult male individuals were analysed:
a) Early/Middle Holocene transition (EMH) (ca. 9-7 ka CAL BP),
b) Early Late Holocene (ELH) (ca. 3.2-1.9 ka. CAL BP),
c) Late Late Holocene (LLH) (ca. 0.9-0.5 ka CAL BP) (Barrientos 1997) (Table 2).

Twelve craniofacial metric variables were selected: OBH (orbital height), OBB (orbital breadth), DKB (interorbital breadth); FMB (bifrontal breadth), ZMB (bizigomaxillary breadth), NLB (nasal breadth), NLH (nasal height), NPH (nasion-prosthion height), ZYB (bizygomatic breadth), WMH (cheek height), MAB (palate breadth, external) (following Howells, 1973), and MAL (maxillo-alveolar length) (following Buikstra and Ubelaker, 1994). Neurocranial variables were omitted from this analysis because the cranial vaults of most specimens were modified, either postdepositionally or culturally. By contrast, the facial skeleton, notwithstanding having experienced fractures and some degree of bone loss, did not suffer plastic alteration or any other significant modification of form. In the present study, the analysis of the variation in both components of form, shape and size, were considered relevant for assessing the degree of differentiation both within and between samples. In order to isolate the shape factor, the raw standardisation of Darroch and Mosimann (1985) was performed. It is based on the calculation, for each individual, of the ratio between each variable and the geometric mean (GM) of all variables (Jungers et al., 1995: 145). The GM was utilised as an overall measure of size. The variations in shape were analysed by means of a bootstrapping discriminant analysis (1,000 resamplings). Prior to the analysis, the samples were tested for normality (Shapiro-Wilks test, $p \leq 0.05$), and homogeneity of variance-covariance (Levene test, $p \leq 0.05$). Due to the small sample sizes, it is not expected that the results of any particular analysis be extremely robust in terms of statistical inference. All that is expected, at this stage of the research, is that they exhibit a relatively high degree of coherence related to the radiocarbon evidence discussed above in order to be accepted as preliminary clues of population change at a regional level.

Results

Radiocarbon data

The probability distribution of the calibrated ^{14}C-ages on a calendar time scale is shown in Figure 2. The emerging pattern is a highly clustered one, which tends to confirm the results of previous analyses performed upon the uncalibrated series (Barrientos, 1997; Barrientos and Perez, 2004a). The four main clusters have an uneven internal distribution of ^{14}C-ages, and are separated from

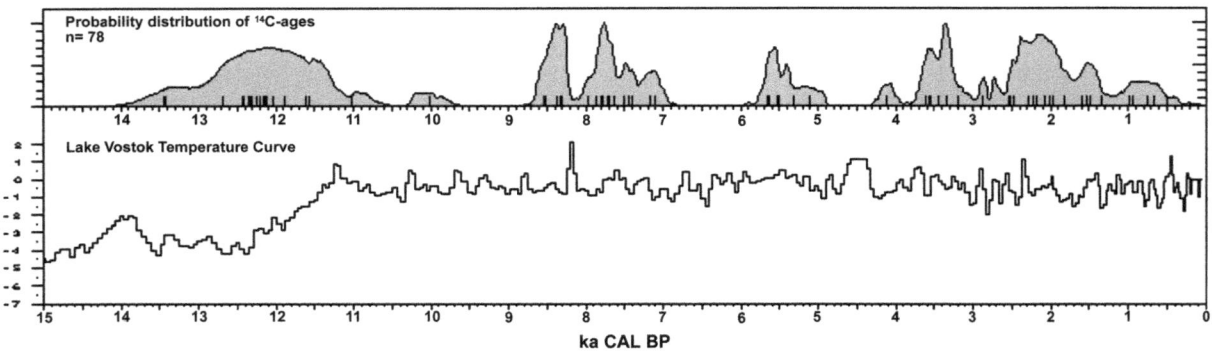

Figure 2. Two-dimensional dispersion calibration figuring showing the probability distribution of the seventy-eight ^{14}C-ages from the southeastern Pampas on the calendar time scale ("calibrated age distribution") (above). Below, the paleotemperature curve from Lake Vostok Ice-Core in east Antarctica.

one another by gaps of differing lengths. This suggests punctuated dynamics of peopling at the regional level.

After the initial colonisation, which occurred during or immediately after the last interstadial of the last glaciation (equivalent to the Allerød of northern Europe; Roberts 1998), there followed a period (ca. 12.5-11.5 ka CAL BP) of seemingly stable occupation of the area during the last stadial (i.e., the Younger Dryas). The archaeological sites from this period are mainly concentrated in hilly environments (Flegenheimer, 1987, 1995; Mazzanti, 1997; Politis and Madrid, 2001), with only a few so far recorded on the plains (Martínez, 1999, 2001; Politis and Madrid, 2001). The intensity of the occupation during the beginnings of the early Holocene seems to have been much lower, with a significant disruption between ca. 9 to 9.5 ka CAL BP.

At about 8.9 ka CAL BP, a new period of intense occupation started, lasting until 6.8 ka CAL BP. The frequency curve representing the distribution of probabilities of the calibrated ^{14}C-ages ages is markedly bimodal, with the interval between the modes coinciding with a major raise in east Antarctica temperatures around 8.2 ka CAL BP. This is probably a southern response to the cold event caused by the shutting down of the thermohaline circulation in the North Atlantic, thereby decreasing thermal transport and resulting in a cold climate persisting in the Northern Hemisphere for several decades (Baldini et al., 2002). This new period of intense occupation of different habitats (e.g., plains, seashore; Politis and Madrid 2001) roughly coincided with the mid-Holocene marine transgression. According to Isla (1989), in our study area, the sea reached its current level at ca. 8000 ^{14}C years BP (i.e., 8.8 ka CAL BP), with peaks around 2.2 to 2.5 m above the current sea level between 6000 and 7000 ^{14}C years BP (ca. 6.8-7.8 ka CAL BP), under predominantly sub-humid to humid conditions. Aguirre and Whatley (1995) date this transgressive event to between 8000 and 6000 ^{14}C years BP (i.e., 8.8-6.8 ka CAL BP), whereas Bonadonna et al. (1995) and Zárate

and Flegenheimer (1991) place it between 6000 and 5000 ^{14}C years BP (i.e., 6.8-5.7 ka CAL BP) (see discussion in Bayón and Politis, 1996).

Between approximately 5 and 4.3 ka CAL BP, there is another major significant gap in the series of calibrated dates (see Barrientos and Perez, 2004a). A similar phenomenon is also recorded in many local sequences in the latitudinal strip situated between 34° and 42° South Lat. (Berón, 1995; Gil, 2000; Sanguinetti de Bórmida and Curzio, 1996), thus constituting a geographically extended, supra-regional pattern. In the southeastern Pampas, it coincides with a warmer-than-today period in east Antarctica, as recorded by the Lake Vostok temperature paleoarchive. At a more local scale, the gap in the radiocarbon record is partially contemporaneous with the post-Hypsithermal climatic worsening and the marine regression period, an event that may be considered as a major ecosystem regulator, affecting both the marine and terrestrial biota of this region (Aguirre and Whatley, 1995; Isla, 1989).

This interval of virtually null evidence of occupation is followed by a relatively short period in which the recorded sites are mainly distributed in plain environments, associated with watercourses and floodplains, and represented by kill/butchering loci of guanaco (*Lama guanicoe*) and other prey mammals (Martínez, 1999; Politis and Madrid, 2001).

At about 4.6-4.4 ka CAL BP there is a minor gap in the calibrated dates series that corresponds to a similar hiatus in the uncalibrated one, which has proved to be non-significant on statistical grounds (Barrientos and Perez, 2004a). It can be interpreted as a consequence of sampling problems rather than of paleodemographic events, although this hypothesis must be carefully tested in the future. After 4.4 ka CAL BP, a continuous albeit multimodal frequency curve of probability distribution of calibrated dates indicates a long period of intense aboriginal occupation of the area lasting until historical times. Coincidentally, most of the sites from this period show evidence indicating that places in the landscape associated with riverine and lagoon environments became the location of residential, multipurpose and long-lasting settlements, frequently used and reused through time (Barrientos et al., 1997; Madrid and Barrientos, 2000; Martínez, 1999, 2002; Martínez and Mackie, 2003; Politis and Madrid, 2001; Politis et al., 2001).

In summary, the temporal distribution of calibrated radiocarbon dates constitutes fairly compelling evidence arguing for a punctuated or discontinuous pattern of occupation of the southeastern Pampas during the Holocene. The fact that the pattern of temporal distribution of the dates is virtually the same as that first reported by Barrientos (1997), despite the addition of 33 new dates to the original dataset (n= 45, representing an increase of 73.3%), strongly suggests that this is a very consistent pattern. Sampling and other largely unknown biases still exist but their contribution to the general picture is probably low.

Morphological data

The first step in the analysis was to assess the degree of differentiation between the diachronic LPSs from the southeastern Pampas. For each individual, the average value of the 1,000 resamplings of the two first canonical scores (100% of the total dispersion) was calculated. The plot of these two scores (Fig. 3) clearly shows that the shape discrimination between the three samples is fairly good (Wilks' lambda Λ=0.016), although the value of the approximate F (1.718; df= 24) is non-significant, probably due to the small sample sizes. The sample that differs the most along the first canonical score, representing 68% of the total dispersion, is that corresponding to the Early/Middle Holocene. Similar results are obtained when the canonical scores (shape) are combined with the GM (size) in a tree clustering analysis using Euclidean distances and the Ward's method as the amalgamation rule (Fig. 3).

Although preliminary, this finding seems to support the claim that the samples derive from at least two, and may be three, different biological populations. These results were those expected under the assumption that the gap in the calibrated radiocarbon dates series observed between 5 and 4.3 ka CAL BP possesses some demographic meaning, possibly reflecting a significant population decrease or a wholesale depopulation after a local extinction occurring during the Mid-Holocene (Barrientos, 1997; Barrientos and Perez, 2004a).

The second step in the analysis was to evaluate the supraregional biological relationships of the diachronic samples of the southeastern Pampas. As there are no samples contemporaneous with that corresponding to the Early/Middle Holocene transition, the comparisons were limited to the Late Holocene (i.e., ca. 3-0.3 ka CAL BP). To accomplish this goal, 14 LPSs deriving from various

different locations in Patagonia (San Blas, Isla Gama, Río Negro, Chubut and Santa Cruz), northeastern Pampas (Paraná Delta), Cuyo (San Juan and Mendoza), and northwestern Argentina (Catamarca) were incorporated into the analysis (Table 2, Fig. 1). Where feasible, these samples were subdivided into subsamples using the presence and type of artificial cranial deformation as the main discriminating criterion. In the Pampas as well as in Patagonia and Cuyo, artificial cranial deformation has proven to be a good temporal indicator, both in relative and absolute terms (Barrientos, 1997, 2001; Baffi and Berón, 1992; Berón and Baffi, 2003; Bórmida, 1953/1954; Novellino et al., 2003), so the type of deformation can be confidently used to estimate the approximate age of a sample (Table 2).

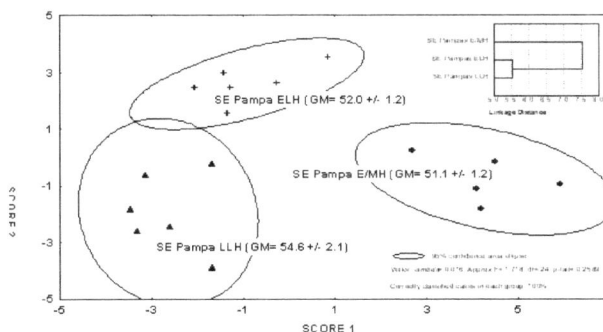

Figure 3. Scatterplot of the average value of 1,000 resamplings of the first two canonical scores (100% of the total dispersion) calculated using 12 transformed (Darroch and Mosimann 1985) craniofacial variables of three diachronic samples from the southeastern Pampas. At the right superior corner, there is a dendrogram resulting from a tree clustering analysis using shape (canonical scores) and size (geometric mean or GM) variables (Euclidean distances and the Ward's method as amalgamation rule).

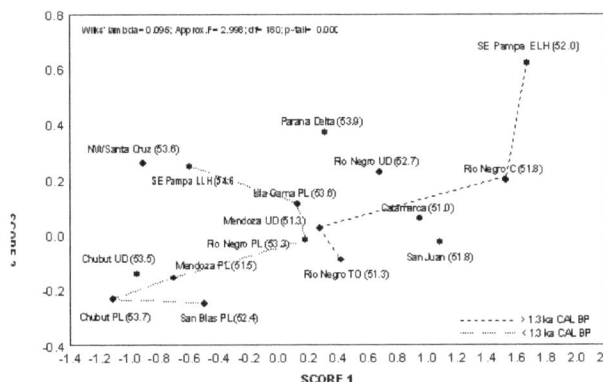

Figure 4. Scatterplot of the average value of 1,000 resamplings of the first two canonical scores (100% of the total dispersion) calculated using 12 transformed craniofacial variables of fourteen samples, showing the biological relationships of the Late Holocene samples of the southeastern Pampas at the supraregional level of analysis (dotted lines).

The statistical procedures were the same as described above except that in this case, the average value of the 1,000 resamplings of the first two canonical scores (55.6% of the total dispersion) was calculated for each sample. Figure 4 is a scatterplot of these two canonical scores. It clearly shows that the samples from the Early and Late Late Holocene of the southeastern Pampas tend to occupy different locations in multivariate space, especially along the first canonical score, and to have different associations with other samples. The sample from the Early Late Holocene of the Pampas is close in shape and size to samples from Río Negro and Mendoza (> 1.3 ka CAL BP), and to more recent samples from San Juan and Catamarca. The sample from the Late Later Holocene of the Pampas is closely related in shape and size to contemporaneous (i.e., < 1.3 ka CAL BP) samples from southwestern (Santa Cruz) and northeastern Patagonia (Chubut, Isla Gama), and, in shape but not in size, to contemporaneous samples from San Blas and Mendoza.

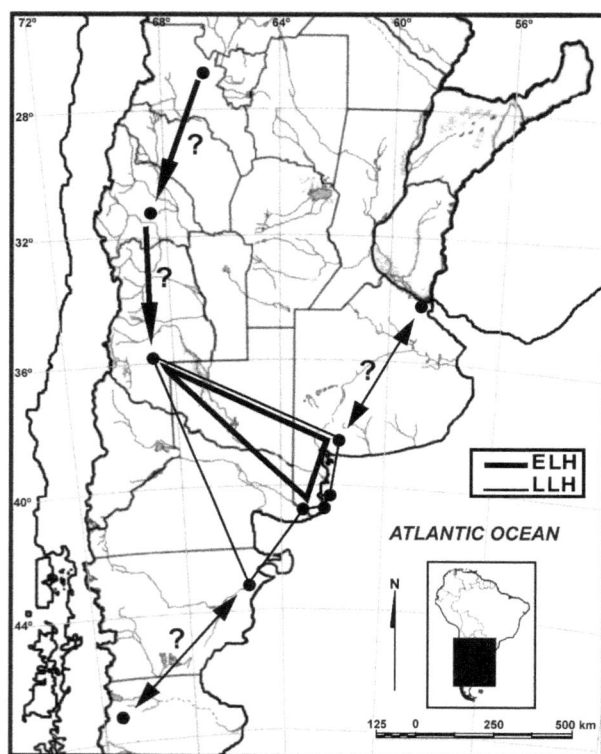

Figure 5. Map showing the hypothesised changing biological relationships of the populations from the southeastern Pampas during the Late Holocene. (ELH = Early Late Holocene, LHH = Late Late Holocene)

These results suggest that the biological influences over the populations of the Pampas changed through time during the Late Holocene. There was first a period in which the local population was closely related to populations from central Argentina (northern Patagonia and Cuyo) and probably also from northwestern Argentina, and a second period, beginning some time after 1.3-1 ka CAL BP, in which the biological relationships of the local population switched to the south, linking it closely with populations from northern and southern Patagonia (Fig. 5). These findings are compatible with the idea advanced in previous papers (Barrientos, 2001; Barrientos and Perez, 2002, 2004b) suggesting a northwards dispersal of populations from northern Patagonia after the Medieval Climatic Anomaly (Stine, 1994), and the subsequent formation of a geographically extensive metapopulation characterised by distinctive biological and cultural traits (e.g., morphology, cranial deformation, mortuary practices, decorative style, economic strategy, etc.).

Discussion

The results presented in this paper, pertaining to two different and independent lines of evidence, clearly show the existence of discontinuities in some aspects of the archaeological and anthropological record of the southeastern Pampas.

On the one hand, the punctuated and clustered distribution of calibrated ^{14}C dates on the calendrical time scale could be interpreted as a probable reflection of past demographic fluctuations. The exact meaning of the gaps between clusters, however, is very difficult to assess at this stage. All that is certain is that some phenomena implying a significant reduction in the archaeological visibility of the local population occurred. Whether these reductions were caused by demographic decline leading to geographic population contraction or by local extinction events remains unclear; this is because the archaeological criteria to distinguish between wholesale depopulation – whatever its cause – from population contraction or shrinkage are not yet fully developed.

On the other hand, the morphological data indicate that different, although probably related, biological populations inhabited the southeastern Pampas during the Holocene, and that population shift followed, in at least one case (i.e. during the Middle Holocene), a significant hiatus in the series of calibrated ^{14}C dates (Barrientos and Perez 2004a).

These two processes, demographic fluctuations (in some cases including both depopulation and local extinction) and population replacement, might cause significant breaks in the evolutionary connection at the population and metapopulation level. The question that immediately arises is, how can this evidence of morphological and demographic discontinuity be reconciled with the notion of cultural continuity represented by the concept of tradition as proposed by previous archaeological models? We are not implying here that biological and cultural evolution should be mechanically linked (a much-discredited notion in anthropology over the last 50 years), but rather are suggesting that any model regarding the local cultural evolution must try to explain cultural continuity in some spheres, not just because of population continuity, but despite biological disruption (cf. Martínez, 2002: 144). Moreover, alternative explanations need to be proposed for the long-lasting, time-transgressive traits that were used to define the archaeological traditions. These persistent traits or patterns of trait association may not necessarily correspond to the "staying power of certain regional-cultural ideas" (Willey, 1945: 56), nor to the secular persistence of rationality patterns relative to the form of producing objects, exploiting resources or sacralising places (Politis and Madrid, 2001: 745). They plausibly reflect constraints to variation imposed by environmental factors such as prey availability and relative abundance, and the mechanical properties of lithic raw materials such as quartzite. In either case, new questions are needed in order to interrogate the archaeological record from a different, and a more evolutionary and paleodemographically oriented perspective.

Conclusions

The hypotheses regarding occupational and populational discontinuities during the Holocene discussed in this paper have yet to be supported by more and higher quality evidence. However, albeit preliminary, our data clearly points to the need to revise some of the premises orient archaeological research in the southeastern Pampas of Argentina. In particular, the belief in the existence of a largely unexplained temporal continuity in rationality patterns mainly represented by technological and economic traits should be evaluated more critically, using different lines of evidence and strategies of research. The one explored here, based in a dialogue between archaeological and bioarchaeological datasets, has proved to be fruitful and encouraging, deserving a further development in a more standardised and systematic way.

Acknowledgements

The authors would like to thank Rafael Goñi for his valuable comments on an earlier version of this paper and Clive Gamble for encouraging the use of calibrated radiocarbon dates in this discussion. This research was made possible thanks to the Fundación Antorchas Research Grant N° 14116-111.

Literature Cited

Aguirre M and Whatley R. 1995. Late Quaternary marginal marine deposits and paleoenvironments from Northeastern Buenos Aires Province, Argentina: A review. *Quaternary Science Review* 14: 223-254.

Ames KM. 2000. Review of the archaeological data. In *Kennewick Man, Cultural Affiliation Report,* Chapter 2.

U.S. Department of Interior, National Park Service, Archaeology and Ethnography Program. http://www.cr.nps.gov/aad/kennewick/ames.htm. Accessed 25/10/2003.

Baffi I and Berón M. 1992. Los restos óseos humanos de Tapera Moreira (La Pampa), y la deformación artificial en la Región Pampeana. Análisis tentativo. *Palimpsesto* 1: 25-36.

Baldini J, McDermott F and Fairchild I. 2002. Structure of the 8200-year cold event revealed by a Speleothem Trace Element Record. *Science* 296: 2203-2206.

Barnard A. 2000. *History and Theory in Anthropology.* Cambridge University Press: Cambridge.

Barrientos G. 1997. *Nutrición y Dieta de las Poblaciones Aborígenes Prehispánicas del Sudeste de la Región Pampeana.* Unpublished Doctoral Dissertation. Facultad de Ciencias Naturales y Museo, UNLP, La Plata.

Barrientos G. 2001. Una aproximación bioarqueológica al estudio del poblamiento prehispánico tardío del Sudeste de la Región Pampeana. *Intersecciones en Antropología* 2: 3-18.

Barrientos G. 2002. The archaeological analysis of death-related behaviors from an evolutionary perspective: Exploring the bioarchaeological record of early American hunter-gatherers. In P*erspectivas Integradoras entre Arqueología y Evolución. Teoría, Método y Casos de Aplicación.,* Martínez G and Lanata JL (eds.). INCUAPA, FACSO, UNICEN: Olavarría; 221-253.

Barrientos G and Perez I. 2002. La dinámica del poblamiento humano del Sudeste de la Región Pampeana durante el Holoceno. *Intersecciones en Antropología* 3: 41-54.

Barrientos G and Perez I. 2004a. Was there a population replacement during the late middle Holocene in the Southeastern Pampas of Argentina? Discussing its archaeological evidence and its paleoecological basis. *Quaternary International.* In press.

Barrientos G and Perez S. 2004b. La expansión y dispersión de poblaciones del norte de Patagonia durante el Holoceno tardío: evidencia arqueológica y modelo explicativo. In *Contra Viento y Marea, Arqueología de la Patagonia.,* Civalero T, Fernandez P and Guraieb G (eds.). Buenos Aires. In press.

Barrientos G, Leipus M and Oliva F. 1997. Investigaciones arqueológicas en la laguna Los Chilenos (Provincia de Buenos Aires). In *Arqueología Pampeana en la Década de los '90.,* Berón M and Politis G (eds.).

Museo de Historia Natural de San Rafael e INCUAPA: San Rafael; 115-125.

Bayon C and Politis G. 1996. Estado actual de las investigaciones en el sitio Monte Hermoso 1. *Arqueología* 6: 83-115.

Berón M. 1995. Cronología radiocarbónica de eventos culturales, y algo más... localidad Tapera Moreira, área del Curacó, La Pampa. *Cuadernos del INAPL* 16: 261-282.

Berón M and Baffi EI. 2003. Procesos de cambio cultural en los cazadores-recolectores de la Provincia de La Pampa, Argentina. *Intersecciones en Antropología* 4: 29-44.

Bocquet-Appel JP and Demars PY. 2000. Neanderthal contraction and modern human colonization of Europe. *Antiquity* 74: 544- 552.

Bonadonna F, Leone G and Zanchetta G. 1995. Composición isotópica de los fósiles de gasterópodos continentales de la provincia de Buenos Aires. Indicaciones paleoclimáticas. In *Evolución Biológica y Climática de la Región Pampeana durante los Últimos Cinco Millones de Años. Un Ensayo de Correlación con el Mediterráneo Occidental.*, Alberdi M, Leone G and Tonni E (eds.). Museo Nacional de Ciencias Naturales, Consejo Superior de Investigaciones Científicas: Madrid; 77-104.

Bórmida M. n.d. *Prolegómenos para una arqueología de la Pampa Bonaerense.* Edición oficial de la provincia de Buenos Aires. Dirección de Bibliotecas, Museos y Archivos Históricos: La Plata.

Bórmida M. 1953/1954. Los antiguos patagones. Estudio de craneología. *Runa* 6: 55-96.

Boschín MT and Llamazares A. 1984. La escuela Histórico-Cultural como factor retardatario del desarrollo científico de la Arqueología Argentina. *Etnía* 32: 101-156.

Boyd R and Richerson P. 1985. *Culture and the Evolutionary Process.* University of Chicago Press: Chicago.

Buikstra J and Ubelaker D. 1994. *Standards for Data Collection from Human Skeletal Remains.* Research Series, no. 44. Arkansas Archaeological Survey: Fayetteville.

Cadien JE, Harris E, Jones W and Mandarino L. 1976. Biological lineages, skeletal populations and microevolution. *Yearbook of Physical Anthropology* 18: 194-201.

Carnese F, Cocilovo J and Goicochea A. 1991/1992. Análisis histórico y estado actual de la antropología biológica en Argentina. *Runa* 20: 35-67.

Cavalli-Sforza LL and Feldman M. 1981. *Cultural transmission and evolution. A quantitative approach.* Princeton University Press: Princeton.

Cronk L, Chagnon N and Irons W. (eds.). 2000. *Adaptation and Human Behavior: An Anthropological Perspective.* Aldine de Gruyter: Hawthorne.

Darroch J and Mosiman J. 1985. Canonical and principal component of shape. *Biometrika* 72: 241-252.

Fix A. 1999. *Migration and Colonization in Human Microevolution.* Cambridge University Press: Cambridge.

Flegenheimer N. 1987. Recent research at localities Cerro La China and Cerro El Sombrero, Argentina. *Current Research in the Pleistocene* 4: 148-149.

Flegenheimer N. 1995. The hill top of Cerro El Sombrero, Argentina. *Current Research in the Pleistocene* 12: 11-13.

Gamble C, Davies W, Pettitt P and Richards M. 2003. Climate change and evolving human diversity in Europe during the last glacial Source. *Philosophical Transactions: Biological Sciences* 359: 243 - 254.

Gil A. 2000. *Arqueología de la Payunia, Provincia de Mendoza.* Unpublished Doctoral Dissertation. Facultad de Ciencias Naturales y Museo, UNLP, La Plata.

Hanski I. 1999. *Metapopulation Ecology.* Oxford University Press: Oxford.

Hanski I and Gilpin M. 1997. *Metapopulation Biology, Ecology, Genetics, and Evolution.* Academic Press: New York.

Housley RA, Gamble CS and Pettitt PB. 2000. Radiocarbon calibration and Lateglacial occupation in northwest Europe: Reply to Blockley et al. *Antiquity* 74: 112-121.

Housley RA, Gamble CS, Street M and Pettitt PB. 1997. Radiocarbon evidence for the Lateglacial human recolonisation of Northern Europe. *Proceedings of the Prehistoric Society* 63: 25-54.

Howells WW. 1973. Cranial Variation in Man. A Study by Multivariate Analysis of Patterns of Difference among Recent Human Populations. Papers of Peabody Museum of Archaeology and Ethnology Vol. 67: Cambridge, Mass.

Imbelloni J. 1938. Tabla clasificatoria de los indios. *Physis* 12: 229-249.

Isla F. 1989. Holocene sea-level fluctuation in the Southern Hemisphere. *Quaternary Science Reviews* 8: 359-368.

Jungers W, Falsetti A and Wall C. 1995. Shape, relative size, and size-adjustments in morphometrics. *Yearbook of Physical Anthropology* 38: 137-161.

Lahr M and Foley R. 1998. Towards a theory of modern human origins: Geography, demography, and diversity in recent human evolution. Yearbook of Physical Anthropology 41: 137-176.

Lahr M. 2002. Extinction in recent human evolution. Abstracts of the IPAM Winter 2002 Conference "Genes, Peoples and Languages". http://www.ipam.ucla.edu/programs/gpl2002/abstracts. Accessed 27/03/2002.

Lande R. 1993. Risks of population extinction from demographic and environmental stochasticity and random catastrophes. *American Naturalist* 142: 911-927.

Lande R, Engen S and Sæther BE. 1998. Extinction times in finite metapopulation models with stochastic local dynamics. *Oikos* 83: 383–389.

Levins R. 1969. Some demographic and genetic consequences of environmental heterogeneity for biological control. *Bulletin of the Entomological Society of America* 15: 237-240.

Liebhold A and Bascompte J. 2003. The Allee effect, stochastic dynamics and the eradication of alien species. *Ecology Letters* 6: 133-140.

Lyman RL, O´Brien MJ and Dunnell RC. 1997. *The Rise and Fall of Culture History.* Plenum Press: New York.

Madrid P and Barrientos G. 2000. La estructura del registro arqueológico del sitio Laguna Tres Reyes 1 (Provincia de Buenos Aires): nuevos datos para la interpretación del poblamiento humano del Sudeste de la Región Pampeana a inicios del Holoceno tardío. *Relaciones de la Sociedad Argentina de Antropología* 25: 179-206.

Martínez G. 1999. *Tecnología, Subsistencia y Asentamiento en el Curso Medio del Río Quequén Grande: Un Enfoque Arqueológico.* Unpublished Doctoral Dissertation. Facultad de Ciencias Naturales y Museo, UNLP, La Plata.

Martínez G. 2001. Archaeological research in Paso Otero 5 site. "Fish-tail" projectile points and megamammals in the Pampean region of Argentina. *Antiquity* 75: 523-528.

Martínez G. 2002. Organización y cambio en las estrategias tecnológicas. Un caso arqueológico e

implicaciones conductuales para la evolución de las sociedades cazadoras-recolectoras Pampeanas. In *Perspectivas Integradoras entre Arqueología y Evolución. Teoría, Métodos Casos de Aplicación.*, Martínez G and Lanata JL (eds.). INCUAPA, FACSO, UNICEN: Olavarría; 121–156.

Martínez G and Mackie Q. 2003. Late Holocene human occupation of the Quequén Grande River valley bottom: Settlement systems and an example of a built environment in the Argentine Pampas. *Before Farming* 4: 1-27.

Masson V, Vimeux F, Jozuel J, Morgan V, Delmotte M, Ciais P, Hammer C, Johnsen S, Lipenkov VY, Mosley-Thompson E, Petit JR, Steig EJ, Stievenard M and Vaikmae R. 2000. Holocene Climate variability in Antarctica Based on 11 Ice-Core Isotopic Records. *Quaternary Research* 54: 348-358.

Mazzanti D. 1997. Archaeology of the Eastern edge of the Tandilia Range (Buenos Aires, Argentina). *Quaternary of South America and Antarctic Peninsula* 10: 211-227.

Menghin O. 1963. Industrias de morfología protolítica en Sudamérica. *Anales de la Universidad del Norte* 2: 69-77.

Menghin O and Bórmida O. 1950. Investigaciones prehistóricas en cuevas de Tandilia (Provincia de Buenos Aires). *Runa* 3: 5-36.

Novellino P, Barrientos G, Perez S, Bernal V and Béguelin M. 2003. Morfometría de las poblaciones humanas tardías del sur de Mendoza. *Revista Argentina de Antropología Biológica* 5: 97.

Parvinen K, Dieckmann U, Gyllenberg M and Metz J. 2003. Evolution of dispersal in metapopulations with local density dependence and demographic stochasticity. *Journal of Evolutionary Biology* 16:143-153.

Petit JR, Jouzel J, Raynaud D, Barkov NI, Barnola JM, Basile I, Bender M, Chappellaz J, Davis J, Delaygue G, Delmonte M, Kotlyakov VM, Legrand M, Lipenkov V, Lorius C, Pépin L, Ritz C, Salzman E and Stievenard M. 1999. Climate and atmospheric history of the past 420 000 years from Vostok ice core, Antarctica. *Nature* 399: 429-436.

Pettitt PB. 2000. Neanderthal extinction: radiocarbon chronology, problems, prospects and an interpretation of the existing data, *Revue d'Archéométrie Supplement. Proceedings of the 3rd International Radiocarbon in Archaeology Conference:* Lyon; 165-77.

Pettitt PB and Pike AWG. 2001. Blind in a cloud of data: problems with the chronology of Neanderthal extinction and anatomically modern human expansion. *Antiquity* 75: 415-420.

Pietrusewsky M. 2000. Metric analysis of skeletal remains: methods and applications. In *Biological Anthropology*. Katzenberg A and Saunders S (eds.). Wiley-Liss: New York; 375-415.

Politis G. 1984. *Arqueología del Area Interserrana Bonaerense*. Unpublished Doctoral Dissertation. Facultad de Ciencias Naturales y Museo, UNLP.

Politis G. 1985. *Cambios climáticos y estrategias adaptativas en el Este de la Región Pampeana (Argentina)*. Paper presented at the 45° Congreso Internacional de Americanistas, Bogotá.

Politis G. 1988a. Paradigmas, modelos y métodos en la arqueología de la pampa bonaerense. *In Arqueología Argentina Contemporánea*, Yacobaccio H (ed.). Búsqueda: Buenos Aires; 59-107.

Politis G. 1988b. Revisión de las unidades de análisis propuestas para representar el cambio cultural en la Región Pampeana. *Precirculados de las Ponencias Científicas Presentadas a los Simposios del IX Congreso Nacional de Arqueología Argentina*: Buenos Aires; 206-218.

Politis G. 1995. The socio-politics of the development of Archaeology in Hispanic South America. In *Theory in Archaeology: A world perspective*, Ucko P (ed.). Routledge: London; 197-235.

Politis G and Madrid P. 2001. Arqueología pampeana: estado actual y perspectivas. In Historia Argentina Prehispánica., Berberian E and Nielsen A (eds.). Editorial Brujas: Córdoba; 737-814.

Politis G, Martinez GA and Bonomo M. 2001. Alfarería temprana en sitios de cazadores recolectores de la Región Pampeana (Argentina). *Latin American Antiquity* 12: 167-181.

Rick JW. 1987. Dates as data: An examination of the Peruvian preceramic radiocarbon record. *American Antiquity* 52: 55-73.

Roberts N. 1998. *The Holocene. An Environmental History*. 2nd Edition. Blackwell Publishers: Oxford.

Sanguinetti de Bórmida A. 1970. La neolitización de las áreas marginales de América del Sur. *Relaciones de la Sociedad Argentina de Antropología* 5: 9-23.

Sanguinetti de Bórmida A and Curzio D. 1996. Cronología regional, cultural y paleoambiental del área de investigación Piedra del Aguila. *Praehistoria* 2: 280-290.

Silveira M.1992. Etnohistoria y arqueología en la Pampa Interserrana (Provincia de Buenos Aires). *Palimpsesto* 2: 29-50.

Smith E and Winterhalder B (eds.). 1992. *Evolutionary Ecology and Human Behavior*. Aldine de Gruyter: Hawthorne.

Sokal R and Crovello T. 1992. The biological species concept: A critical evaluation. In *The Units of Evolution. Essays on the Nature of Species*, Ereshefsky M. (ed.). The MIT Press: Cambridge; 27-55.

Stine S. 1994. Extreme and persistent drought in California and Patagonia during mediaeval time. *Nature* 369: 546-549.

Van Vark G and Schaasfma W. 1992. Advances in quantitative analysis of skeletal morphology. In *Skeletal Biology of Past Peoples: Research Methods*, Saunders S and Katzemberg A (eds.). Willey-Liss: New York; 225-257.

Weninger B. 1997. *Studien zur dendrochronologischen Kalibration von archäologischen ^{14}C-Daten*. Habelt Verlag: Frankfurt.

Weninger B, Jöris O and Danzeglocke U. 2003. Cologne Radiocarbon Calibration & Palaeoclimate Research Package. http://www.calpal.de. Accessed 25/09/03.

Willey GR. 1945. Horizon styles and pottery traditions in Peruvian archaeology. *American Antiquity* 10: 49-56.

Willey GR and Phillips P. 1958. *Method and Theory in American Archaeology*. University of Chicago Press: Chicago.

Willey GR and Sabloff JA. 1980. *A History of American Archaeology*, 2nd. ed. Freeman: San Francisco.

Zárate M and Flegenheimer N. 1991. Geoarchaeology of the Cerro La China Locality (Buenos Aires, Argentina): Site 2 and Site 3. *Geoarchaeology: An International Journal* 6: 273-294.

Measuring variation in the Neolithic human bones from the Orkney Islands

Neolithic Orcadian Diversity

John Bernal*, Sonia Zakrzewski & Andrew Jones

Dept of Archaeology, University of Southampton
Highfield, Southampton, SO17 1BF
* e-mail address for correspondence: jab202@soton.ac.uk

Abstract

Human skeletal remains from the Orkney Island Neolithic tombs (4500 – 5500 BP) were examined in order to identify statistically significant differences in metric and non-metric variation within and between the tomb populations. If the burial populations of the Orkneys represented heterogeneous groups, then the skeletal material could be expected to exhibit statistically significant differences between tombs. If homogeneous, then the skeletal material would likely exhibit few differences.

Statistically significant differences in some cranial measurements were identified between the burial populations. The variation found was likely to be due to genetic drift, as found within any homogeneous population, and thus was not an unusual amount of craniometric variation. Such differences would be reasonably likely to occur within tomb populations when those tombs were in continuous for over 800 to 1000 years. The cranial measurements suggest a reasonably homogeneous population.

Statistical analysis, however, identified significant differences in the upper second molar crown width between the Quanterness burial population and other Orkney burial populations. Unlike cranial measurements, genetic drift would not likely explain the statistically significant difference in crown width. Such a difference could be representative of a population at Quanterness that was biologically distinct in some way from the other groups.

Keywords: population history, human diversity, craniometrics, Neolithic, Orkney Islands, teeth

Introduction

The Orkney Islands, located approximately 16 kilometres off the northeast coast of Scotland, have yielded many burials from chambered tombs dated to the Neolithic (Fig. 1). Radiocarbon dates for some of the bones, as described by Renfrew (1985) and Barber (1997), suggest continuous use of the tombs throughout the early and middle Neolithic (4500-5500 BP). Most Orcadian skeletal reports written over the past 150 years (Garson 1884; Charleson 1902; Low 1934, 1935, 1936; Wells 1951; Renfrew 1979; Chesterman 1983; Barber 1997) have primarily dealt with material from individual sites. Few reports have included any cross comparative analysis of the skeletal material, and none of the reports have analysed systematically the skeletal material in order to identify statistically significant variation between tomb populations. This study assessed the available human skeletal material for statistically significant variation between and within the tomb populations.

The island population of Neolithic Orkney may have represented either a relatively isolated homogeneous population or a population consisting of several heterogeneous groups. If homogeneous, then the skeletal material would be expected to exhibit little significant

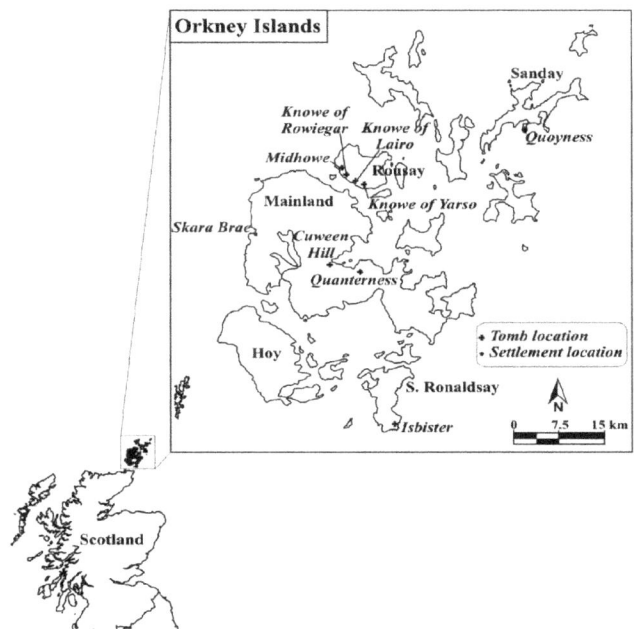

Figure 1. Map of Orkney Islands with site locations.

variation, perhaps even indications of familial traits within individual tombs. If heterogeneous, then the skeletal material would be expected to exhibit significant variation between tombs. As Buikstra and Ubelaker (1994, 69) note, "population variation in skeletal morphology is the result of genetic and environmental influences." Gene flow and natural selection play a primary role in the heritability of skeletal morphology among groups. Any statistically significant difference between groups could provide evidence of group homogeneity or heterogeneity within Neolithic Orkney populations.

Conversely, factors other than genetics can influence skeletal morphology and must be taken into account for reliability purposes. Age, sex, activity patterns, diet, disease, and environmental conditions may also have an effect on bone development. However, it is likely that environmental conditions, activity patterns, diet, and disease load would not be significantly different in such a confined regional area as the Orkney Islands. Genetic influence, therefore, would remain the most likely explanation of any significant differences within the Orkney populations.

The vast majority of skeletal material recovered from the sites was commingled and in various states of preservation. Taphonomic processes certainly have had an impact on bone preservation, but the extent cannot be easily ascertained. Additionally, subsequent disturbance of the sites since the Neolithic including modern excavation and recovery bias may have had some effect on the preservation and distribution of bone.

The degree to which burial practices may have had an effect on the condition and distribution of bone from each site is not known. The issue raises the further possibility that bones were not only commingled within individual tombs but also commingled between tombs (Reilly, 2003). Such burial practice as moving bones between tombs is a concern and would have a great impact upon the results of this study. This impact would be the greatest on comparisons between tombs but would not have an effect on the population analysed as a whole. The potential of bone dispersal throughout the tombs is not known. Therefore, the reasonable assumption prior to analysis was that the tomb populations could at least provide a crude representation of the living population as a whole.

Other potential problems associated with the study of burial populations are based on the questionable reliability of burials as being representative of living populations. The osteological paradox recognizes a major problem associated with interpretations based on skeletal material (Wood et al. 1992:345). Direct demographic profiles cannot be obtained, as burial samples are biased, in that not all individuals are represented for a variety of reasons. There is no way of knowing all of the factors that would have influenced the makeup of the burial population. The current study did not find a significant bias in age or sex distribution in most tombs, as both sexes and all age ranges were well represented. Such representation indicates that a bias in male-female or young-old burials was not present.

Materials and Methods

Only adult specimens were measured and used for comparison, as significant changes in *normal* healthy bone ceases upon reaching adulthood. All of the skeletal material analysed in this report (Table 1) was recovered from the Neolithic sites at Cuween Hill, Isbister, Knowe of Rowiegar, Knowe of Yarso, Midhowe, Quanterness, Quoyness, and Skara Brae.

Table 1. Summary of Orkney Island sites, bones and sample size used in this study.

Site	Bone					
	skull	humerus	femur	tibia	radius	ulna
Cuween Hill	6	-	-	-	-	-
Isbister	21	16	15	14	5	1
Papa Westray	2	-	1	-	-	-
Knowe of Rowiegar	2	2	1	4	1	3
Knowe of Yarso	4	-	1	-	-	-
Midhowe	-	5	2	4	-	1
Quanterness	1	3	1	1	13	8
Quoyness	-	1	-	-	-	-
Skara Brae	-	2	2	2	2	-
Total n	36	29	23	25	21	13

The skeletal collections used in this study are located at the National Museum of Scotland in Edinburgh, the Marischal Museum at the University of Aberdeen, and the Tankerness Museum in Kirkwall, Orkney.

All of the data collected was entered into a Microsoft Access 2000 database and exported to Microsoft Excel 2000 and SPSS (Version 11.5) in order to conduct statistical analyses. The limited sample size required the pooling of sexes and sites for comparative purposes. Analyses included linear regression models and one-way analysis of variance (ANOVA) to identify significant differences defined as $p \leq 0.05$.

As the Orkney material was commingled and lacked associated sexually dimorphic elements, such as the pelvis, the accuracy rate of sex determination for individual skull and long bones was subject to error in ambiguous cases. Unfortunately, no practical means exists by which to verify the sex of each specimen. However, the data was carefully reviewed in any ambiguous case, but should always be considered to be 'best estimates' rather than 'certainties'.

Cranial Methods

Estimation of age and determination of sex were based on methods described by Buikstra and Ubelaker (1994). Estimation of age was determined by cranial suture closure, sphenooccipital synchondrosis fusion, third molar eruption, and/or tooth wear (Brothwell 1981).

Determination of sex involved the ranking of sexually dimorphic traits including development of the nuchal crest, mastoid process, supra-orbital margin, and supra-orbital ridge. Additionally, the mental eminence, gonial flaring, robusticity, and squareness of the mandible were also used when available.

Direct cranial measurements were taken following Howells (1973). Measurements were chosen on the basis of those most frequently used for comparative purposes and the ease with which they could be repeated with minimal error. In a few cases, involving slightly damaged skulls, measurements were estimated if it was felt that this method would be reasonably precise. Data for skulls not available for direct study (i.e. lost from collections) was obtained from the original reports. This data must be considered as questionable as it is not known whether the same measurement techniques were used. In order to reduce this uncertainty, measurements for all available skulls were taken and compared with the data from the original reports. All were found to be within ±3 mm. It can thus be reasonably assumed that the measurements for lost or missing skulls could be reliably obtained from the original reports. Although skulls from the Isbister collection were available for analysis, it was decided that only two skulls, representing 10% of the Isbister collection, would be measured and compared with original measurements from Chesterman (1983). As the measurements directly taken were within ±2 mm of those recorded by Chesterman, the remaining Isbister skulls were not directly re-measured. Chesterman's original measurements therefore were used in order to avoid repeating data collection. A total of 36 skulls were examined, of which 30 skulls (23 male and 7 female) were included in the final analysis. Six skulls were excluded from the final data set due to pathology, damage, or non-adult status.

Cranial indices, as described in Bass (1995), were used to express ratios or relationships of cranial variables for comparative purposes. Cranial indices are presented in

percentages and define skulls into ranges on the basis of raw shape. The indices are ratios or relationships of two combined dimensions of the skull such as length and height. Cranial non-metric traits were also recorded, following Berry & Berry (1967).

Cranial variables were checked for normal distribution with P-P plots and histograms. One cranial variable maxilla-alveolar breadth (MAB) was not used, due to its non-normal distribution of measurement values; this is most likely due to differential methods in measurement techniques. All other variables were normally distributed.

Postcranial methods

Postcranial measurements were taken following Buikstra and Ubelaker (1994). Determination of sex was based on maximum length and general robusticity (i.e. anterior-posterior measurements). However, as many of the postcranial bones were commingled, the determination of sex could not be stated with a high degree of confidence. For the Isbister bones and lost specimens, data for the humerus and femur, including length and determination of sex, was indirectly obtained from the original skeletal reports. Postcranial non-metric trait data was recorded following Finnegan (1978).

Due to the limited size of the sample, both left and right specimens were included in all data analyses. In a few cases, this involved paired long bones from the same individual. As the material was commingled we cannot know how many other times paired bones from the same individual occur within the sample, and thus all bones were included in analyses. Sites were pooled in order to conduct statistical analyses. Such pooling decisions were based solely on the maximum number of reliable data samples that could be provided and is noted in the analysis and results. Stature comparisons were not conducted due to the questionable reliability of sex determination based upon postcranial bones and the high standard errors associated with stature formulae.

Dental methods

Dental wear, caries, hypoplasia, and tooth measurements were recorded for each specimen, but only adult molar teeth were used for comparative analysis. Molars were divided into upper and lower first, second, and third molars, and both left and right antimeres were included in analysis. Each molar was measured to the nearest 0.1 mm with digital callipers. Maximum crown length / mesio-distal diameter (ML) and maximum crown width / bucco-lingual diameter (BL) was measured, following Buikstra & Ubelaker (1994). Although diameter was measured on all molars, only the second molar (n = 123) was used in analysis. Wear (1st molars) and extreme size variation (3rd molars) made the measurements taken upon these molars unreliable and unsuitable for analysis.

Results

Craniometrics

Sexual dimorphism between the Orkney sexes was examined. There were statistically significant differences in cranial length (GOL) at $p < 0.001$ (n = 28), basion-nasion length (BNL) at $p = 0.048$ (n = 21), facial length (BPL) at $p = 0.010$ (n = 18), and upper facial height (NPH) at $p = 0.037$ (n = 19) between the determined sexes. In each of the above measurements, as expected, skulls determined as male were statistically larger in size. When cranial length (GOL), basion-nasion length (BPL), and upper facial height (NPH) were plotted, cluster analysis showed sexual dimorphism between the sexes more clearly (Fig. 2), although the sample size for estimated females was limited.

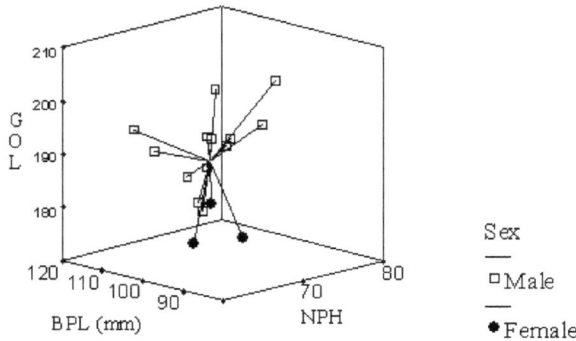

Figure 2. The sexual dimorphism between male (n = 13) and female (n = 3) in facial (BPL), cranial (GOL) lengths, and upper facial (NPH) height.

As the Isbister sample was the largest in number, variation between the Orkney tombs was examined by comparing the Isbister sample with a pooled sample of all other Orkney tomb populations. Significant differences in cranial measurements and cranial indices were identified between the two groups, and are described below.

Cranial height (BBH)

One-way analysis of variance (ANOVA) indicated significant differences between the two groups in cranial height (BBH) at $p = 0.003$ (n = 23). The strength of the relationship between the observed and model-predicted values of BBH was fairly strong ($R = 0.584$). According to the linear model only 34% of the variation in BBH could be accounted for in terms of intra site variation ($R^2 = 0.341$). The Isbister mean BBH (136 mm, n = 12) is significantly greater than that obtained from the pooled sites (131 mm, n = 11) (Fig. 3).

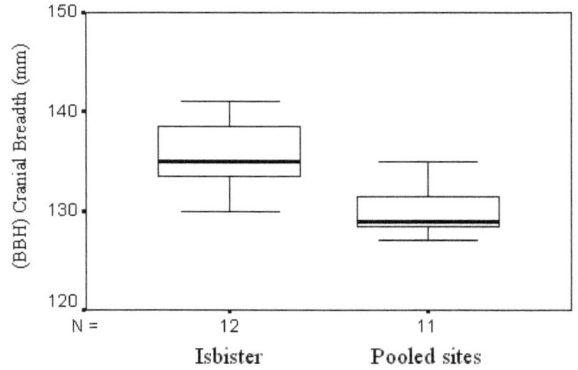

Figure 3. The significant variation between the Isbister site (n = 12) and the pooled sites (n = 11) in mean cranial height (BBH) at $p = 0.003$, sexes pooled.

Facial prognathism (BPL)

ANOVA indicated significant differences between the two groups in facial prognathism (BPL) at $p = 0.015$. A relationship between the observed and model-predicted values of BPL was fairly strong ($R = 0.561$, $R^2 = 0.315$). The BPL mean calculated from the pooled sites (105 mm, n = 7) is significantly greater than that from the Isbister sample (97 mm, n = 11) (Fig. 4).

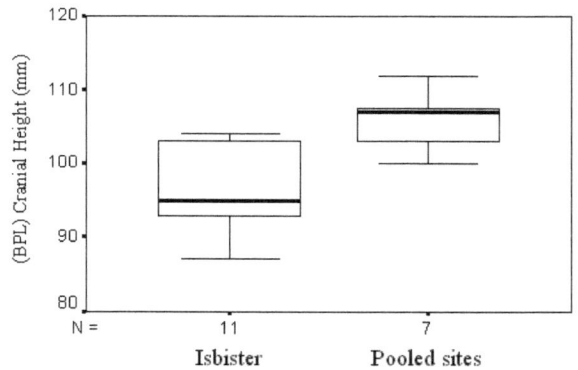

Figure 4. The significant variation between the Isbister site (n = 11) and the pooled sites (n = 7) in the mean facial prognathism (BPL) at $p = 0.015$, sexes pooled.

Cranial length-height index (LHI)

ANOVA indicated significant differences between the two groups in the mean length-height index (LHI) at $p = 0.045$ (n = 22, $R = 0.432$, $R^2 = 0.187$). The Isbister mean LHI (72 mm, n = 11) is significantly greater than that from the pooled sites (69 mm, n = 11) (Fig. 5).

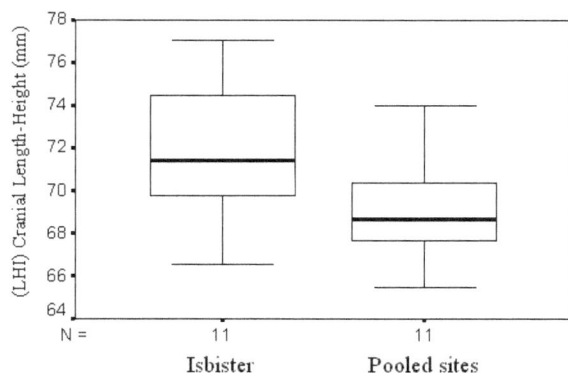

Figure 5. The significant variation between the Isbister site (n = 11) and the pooled sites (n = 11) in the cranial length-height (LHI) at p = 0.045, sexes pooled.

Postcranial analysis

No significant differences within or between the tomb populations were found in any of the postcranial measurements. It would have been unusual, however, to find significant differences in measurements between tomb populations, as, the factors influencing postcranial bone development in the Orkney region are likely to have been the same on a population level. Significant differences, therefore, in postcranial development, beyond sexual dimorphism, are unlikely to exist between these populations.

The high degree of overlap in bone measurements between the sexes suggests that original determination of sex for postcranial bones may be incorrect in some cases or that there is little sexual dimorphism in these groups. This is likely to be due to the commingled state of the Orcadian material and the difficulty involved in determining the sex of individual long bone specimens. Both sexes in Orkney were very robust and the degree of sexual dimorphism, based on gross visual examination, was low. Wells (1951) has previously shown that difficulties exist in sex determination in these populations (specifically within the Quoyness sample).

Dental analysis

One-way analysis of variance (ANOVA) showed a significant difference between the sites at Papa Westray (n = 6), Quanterness (n = 20), Rowiegar (n = 10), and Yarso (n = 2) in the crown width diameter or bucco-lingual (BL) diameter for upper second molars (p = 0.009).

Due to the minute level at which tooth measurements were made (±0.1mm), caution was taken in accepting the difference found in the crown width diameter (BL). The data set was reviewed, and, on the basis of raw measurements, five ambiguous and unusual molars were found and removed from the data set. Even with removal

of those particular molars, a significant difference was still observed. The data set was therefore again reviewed to identify any potential errors in the recording or identification of these specimens, as it was thought possible that these five questionable molars might have been identified incorrectly or that they might have derived from young individuals. In one case, the molar was in occlusion in an intact adult maxilla from the site of Papa Westray, indicating that neither age nor misidentification was a factor. The remaining four molars, from Quanterness, also derived from adult jaws as three of the four had adulthood wear stages (grades 3+ to 4) (Brothwell 1981). It was concluded that neither misidentification nor age were likely to have caused an error and the questionable molars were subsequently placed back into the data set.

Errors in measurement technique may have led to this difference. The Quanterness sample was the first group measured and intra-observer repetition error may have taken place as a result. If such a methodological error were made, similar errors would also be expected in other dental measurements, such as crown length. No significant difference in the crown length was found. Instrument error was also considered to be unlikely as the same set of callipers was used for all measurements. It was thus determined that recording error did not account for the significant difference between sites, and thus the significant difference in BL diameter is probably real.

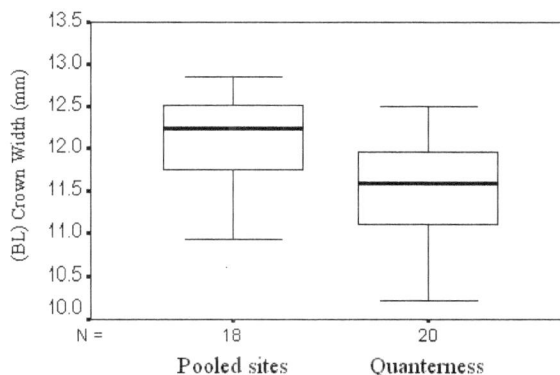

Figure 6. The significant variation between the pooled sites (n = 18) and the Quanterness site (n = 20) in the crown width (BL) of the upper second molar at p = 0.001.

ANOVA tests were run between all the groups to verify the difference. Based upon the post-hoc tests, Quanterness was confirmed as the statistically significantly different group. The Quanterness group (n = 20) was then compared to the other sites pooled together (n = 18). ANOVA found a significant difference in the BL crown width (p = 0.001). The strength of the relationship between the observed and model-predicted values was fairly strong ($R = 0.508$), however, only 26% of the variation could be accounted for in terms of site difference ($R^2 = 0.258$).

Figure 6 shows the variation more clearly, with the Quanterness mean crown width (11.5 mm, n = 20) significantly lower than the pooled sites (12.1 mm, n = 18). No significant differences were found in other teeth.

Discussion

How much variation would be required to distinguish between distinct Orkney burial populations? Larsen (1997, 302) argues that an unusually high frequency of variation in measurements would be required to make a distinction between groups. Three statistically significant differences in cranial measurements exist between Isbister and the other tomb populations. This is neither high nor low. It is possible that the female group could have a significant impact on the results had the group been weighted in either the Isbister or the pooled tombs data set. However, this possibility was checked by univariate analysis of variance, with no significant impact identified. The estimated females were evenly distributed between the two groups. Initially, it was tempting to attribute the statistically significant differences in measurement results to real genetic differences between groups. Additional analysis, however, based upon other populations, showed that statistically significant variation in three cranial measurements within a homogenous population is common.

Comparisons were also made between the Orcadian crania and the Howells (1973) global craniometric series, in order to identify the morphologically most similar population to the Orkney group. The Hungarian Zalavár were the morphologically closest group based on comparison of all cranial measurements, as the Zalavár had the fewest statistically significant differences from the entire Orkney skeletal data set used in the current study. Ten different subgroups from within the Zalavár population were created. Each subgroup contained a random selection of the same number of skulls and male to female ratio as the Orkney population. Each of these ten Zalavár subgroups was randomly set up in the same exact site to sex ratio as the Orkney sample. ANOVA was run on each of the ten groups in the same manner as the Orkney skulls in order to identify patterns in significant differences, if any. As expected, significant differences were found between the sexes in each of the groups to varying degrees. The population within each group was then randomly pooled into two separate groups. In seven of the ten groups, significant differences of between one and four cranial measurements were found. The three remaining groups had no significant differences. The results of this mini test showed that the significant differences within the Orkney population would also occur in other homogeneous populations. Therefore, the simplest and most likely explanation of the significant differences found within the Orkney population may be attributed to normal genetic drift, as would occur in any similar population continuously burying its dead in the same tombs for 800 to 1000 years.

Dental variation was also seen within the sample. The Quanterness tomb population had a lower mean diameter in upper second molar BL crown width. A linear regression model could only attribute 25% of the variation to intra-site difference. The remaining 75% of the variance could be attributed to any number of factors. This is intriguing in that the sample for Quanterness contained a minimum number of individuals (MNI) of 10 and the pooled sites MNI = 9, indicating that the difference is unlikely to be the result of sexual dimorphism. For the difference to be the result of sexual dimorphism, all or most of the Quanterness teeth (MNI = 10) would have to be from one sex and all or most of the pooled group teeth (MNI = 9) from the other sex. It would also have to assume that statistically significant sexual dimorphism exists in M^2 BL crown width. Unfortunately there was no way to distinguish between Orkney male and female teeth. Nevertheless, it is unlikely that all of these conditions would coincide to explain the difference observed.

Diet, dental wear and/or disease could have had an effect on the development of the Quanterness teeth, and thus explain the difference in crown width. The population may have experienced some form of dietary and/or disease stress during childhood that caused developmental differences in crown width. This argument would require the Quanterness population (MNI =10) to be contemporaneous in order to experience the same level of stress. Again, it is difficult to imagine such conditions occurring, and therefore this does not appear to explain the difference in crown width. A complete lack of dental caries and hypoplasia from the teeth at Quanterness do not indicate differences between the samples in terms of diet or level of stress. Dental wear generally affects the mesio-distal diameter (ML) to a much greater extent than the BL measurement (Hillson 1996), and hence is also unlikely to account for the size difference seen.

Heritability of crown diameters is observed in modern populations (Hillson, 1996), and hence genetic factors appear the most likely explanation for the differences in BL crown width between the groups. The differences observed in the upper second molar may be evidence of group distinction at the Quanterness site. The Quanterness burials may represent a group that was much more closely related than other Orkney groups. The Neolithic populations of Orkney may not have interacted and interbred with all groups to the same degree. For example, groups may have been more inclined to form close relationships with those living on the same islands. Alternatively, period(s) of conflict between groups within the same island may have influenced relationships with other island groups, thereby potentially increasing contact with other island populations. This may also explain the disparity in the MNI reported between Quanterness and the other tombs, with the exception of Isbister (Garson

1884; Charleson 1902; Low 1934, 1935, 1936; Wells 1951; Renfrew 1979; Chesterman 1983; Barber 1997). The Quanterness group therefore may have been a distinct group with distinctly different burial practices. Unfortunately, due to time constraints, the teeth from the Isbister sample could not be measured. Additional archaeological evidence would be required to confirm such a conclusion.

Although evidence is lacking, it is hardly unreasonable to predict that familial relationships occurred within the tomb populations. To what extent it may have occurred remains unknown. It was initially hoped that evidence of familial relationships, if any, could be identified in the skeletal remains. Specifically, it had been hoped that non-metric traits, both cranial and postcranial, could provide an answer. Unfortunately, no evidence was identified to support familial relationships, though the limited sample size and condition of the bones restricted the amount of information that could be gained in this area.

Conclusion

The observed cranial variation between Orkney burial populations was likely due to genetic drift, as would be found within any homogeneous population. Given that the tombs were in continuous use over 800 to 1000 years, it may be reasonably assumed that the tomb burials were not all contemporaneous. Such morphological differences therefore would be even more likely to occur in this type of skeletal population sample. The results of the craniometric analyses in this study therefore suggest a homogeneous Orcadian population during the Neolithic period.

Nevertheless, biologically distinct groups within Orkney cannot be ruled out, as statistical analysis did find significant differences in the upper second molar crown width between the Quanterness burial population and the other Orkney burial populations. Unlike cranial measurements, genetic drift likely would not explain the statistically significant difference in crown width. Such a difference could be representative of a population at Quanterness that was biologically distinct in some way from the other groups. Tooth size is a heritable trait that remains relatively stable in modern populations (Hillson, 1996), and hence variation in molar tooth size would not be expected within a homogeneous population. There is little chance that sexual dimorphism can explain the difference in crown width at Quanterness, and thus, the variation is likely due to biological differences.

This study has attempted to define the Orkney tomb populations in terms of a homogeneous group or as several heterogeneous groups. In some respects this has been accomplished. It is, however, likely that many different modes of interaction between groups were taking place in Neolithic Orkney. Populations are not static and change is inevitable. The factors that influence change in populations are many and skeletal remains may or may not reflect those changes. Future analysis of the Orkney bones will continue to expand our information about the Orkney inhabitants, as the human bones from Orkney comprise one of the best skeletal collections from the Neolithic. Further comparison with other British Neolithic skeletal remains is warranted. Garson (1884) published a thorough account of some of the first Orkney bones recovered from Skara Brae. More than a century later the Orkney bones are still being studied. It is also hoped that well beyond a century from now the Orkney bones will continue to be examined and yield valuable information.

Acknowledgements

The authors would like to thank Anne Brundle (Tankerness Museum, Orkney), Dr Neil Curtis (Marischal Museum, Aberdeen), Dr Alison Sheridan (National Museum of Scotland), and Daphne Lorrimer (Mainland, Orkney) for their time and for providing access to the Orkney Islands skeletal material. Partial funding for this project was obtained from the Department of Archaeology (University of Southampton).

Literature Cited

Barber J (1997) *The Excavation of a Stalled Cairn at the Point of Cott, Westray, Orkney.* Edinburgh: Scottish Trust for Archaeological Research.

Bass WM (1995) *Human Osteology: A Laboratory and Field Manual* (Fourth edition). Columbia, Missouri: Missouri Archaeological Society.

Berry AC and Berry RJ (1967) Epigenetic Variation in the Human Cranium. *Journal of Anatomy* 101(2): 361-379.

Brothwell DR (1981) *Digging up Bones: The Excavation, Treatment, and Study of Human Skeletal Remains.* London: British Museum.

Buikstra JE and Ubelaker DH (1994) S*tandards for Skeletal Collection from Human Skeletal Remains.* Fayetteville: Arkansas Archaeological Survey Research Series No. 44.

Charleson MM (1902) Notice of a Chambered Cairn in the Parish of Firth, Orkney. *Proceedings of the Society of Antiquaries of Scotland* 36: 733-738.

Chesterman JD (1983) The Human Skeletal Remains. In JW Hedges (ed.): *Isbister: A Chambered Tomb in Orkney.* Oxford: BAR Publishing. BAR British Series 115: 73-132.

Finnegan M (1978) Non-Metric Variation of the Infracranial Skeleton. *Journal of Anatomy* 125(1): 23-37.

Garson JG (1884) On the Osteology of the Ancient Inhabitants of the Orkney Islands. *The Journal of the Anthropological Institute of Great Britain and Ireland* XIII: 54-86.

Hillson S. (1996) *Dental Anthropology*. Cambridge, Cambridge University Press.

Howells WW (1973) Cranial Variation in Man: A Study of Multivariate Analysis of Patterns of Difference Among Recent Human Populations. *Papers of the Peabody Museum of Archaeology and Ethnology* 67: 1-259.

Larsen CS (1997) *Bioarchaeology: Interpreting Behavior from the Human Skeleton.* Cambrige: Cambridge University Press.

Low A (1934) Description of the Human Skeletal Remains. In JG Callander and WG Grant (eds): A Long Stalled Chambered Cairn or Mausoleum (Rousay type) near Midhowe, Rousay, Orkney. *Proceedings of the Society of Antiquaries of Scotland* 68: 343-348.

Low A (1935) Report on the Human Skeletal Remains. In JG Callander and WG Grant (eds): A Long Stalled Cairn, the Knowe of Yarso, Orkney. *Proceedings of the Society of Antiquaries of Scotland* 69: 344-351.

Low A (1936) Report on the Human Bones from the Knowe of Ramsey, Rousay, Orkney. In JG Callander and WG Grant (eds): A Stalled Chambered Cairn, Knowe of Ramsay, at Hullion, Rousay, Orkney. *Proceedings of the Society of Antiquaries of Scotland* 70: 414-414.

Reilly S (2003) Processing the Dead in Neolithic Orkney. *Oxford Journal of Archaeology* 22(2): 133-154.

Renfrew C (1979) *Investigations in Orkney*. London: Society of Antiquaries of London.

Renfrew C (1985) *The Prehistory of Orkney*. Edinburgh: Edinburgh University Press.

Wells LH (1951) Note on the Human Skeletal Fragments from the Quoyness Cairn. In VG Childe (ed.): Re-excavation of the Chambered Cairn of Quoyness, Sanday, on Behalf of the Ministry of Works in 1951-2. *Proceedings of the Society of Antiquaries of Scotland* 86: 137-138.

Wood JW, Milner GR, Harpending HC, and Weiss KM (1992) The Osteological Paradox: Problems of Inferring Prehistoric Health from Skeletal Samples. *Current Anthropology* 33(4): 343-370.

Fluctuating Asymmetry: A Potential Osteological Application

Fluctuating Asymmetry

Rebecca A. Storm* and Christopher J. Knüsel

Biological Anthropology Research Centre (BARC)
Department of Archaeological Sciences, University of Bradford
Bradford
West Yorkshire
BD7 1DP

* e-mail address for correspondence: storm333@supanet.com

Abstract

Fluctuating, directional and anti-asymmetry are three forms of biological asymmetry found in the human skeleton. Of these, fluctuating asymmetry is the most effective in the detection of osseous changes influenced by biomechanics, genetics, pathology, and environmental stress. The objective of the current study is to create a database of these skeletal asymmetries from 128 measurements of the cranial and postcranial skeleton (the cranium, mandible, clavicle, scapula, humerus, radius, ulna, metacarpals, sacrum, *os coxae*, femur, tibia, calcaneus, talus and the 1st metatarsal) so as to evaluate the uses of fluctuating asymmetry in physical anthropology and to highlight the consequences of ignoring such asymmetries in standard osteological research. By using these measurements to determine the existence and extent of fluctuating asymmetry it is possible to infer handedness, congenital abnormalities, disease, sexual diversity, and evolutionary changes in skeletal material. Once these inferences have been made about the individual, further suppositions can be formulated about the population as a whole, including social structures, health indices, genetic patterning, and environmental and living conditions. This paper focuses on the analysis of 17 cranial and mandibular measurements applied to a small sample of two medieval populations, Hickeleton and Chichester. One individual, Chichester skeleton 32, was found to deviate strongly from the population norm. Differential diagnosis indicates a possible case of either muscular torticollis or the result of biomechanical stress not exhibited in the others within the population. From this diagnosis further inferences can be made both of individual's and of the population's life experiences. Chichester 32 thus demonstrates the potential usefulness of the larger study of fluctuating asymmetry in skeletal populations.

Key Words: Fluctuating asymmetry, congenital abnormalities, torticollis.

Introduction

There are three main types of asymmetry found in bilateral structures such as the human skeleton. These are directional asymmetries, anti-symmetries, and fluctuating asymmetries. Directional asymmetry, also known as fixed or differentiated-directional asymmetry, occurs when the bone development of one side of a skeleton is favoured over the other. Anti-symmetry occurs when asymmetry is present but varies in which side it predominantly occurs (Fields et al.1995; Steele & Mays 1995; Dittmar 1998; Albert & Greene 1999; Storm 2000). Fluctuating asymmetry is variation in the right and left sides of a bilateral structure. These variations are random, independent and usually the differences are small, less than 1% of the measurable trait (Van Valen 1962; Palmer 1994). In a bilateral structure, the normal process of development is the creation of an exact mirror image of each side of the structure, thus creating perfect symmetry. However, once this is development is disrupted, fluctuating asymmetry occurs (Larsen 1997). This disruption is caused by variation in the environment of the developing structure and is usually termed biological or developmental noise. If it is postulated that the greater the development stability, the greater the symmetry, then the hypothesis can be made that any movement away from symmetry reflects environmental and biological instability which can thus be measured (Palmer 1994; Fields et al. 1995; McManus 2002).

Of the three categories of asymmetry, fluctuating asymmetry is of most potential interest in osteological studies. Unlike some studies that record morphological variation based solely on descriptions, which can be limited and subjective, the purpose of the current study is to demonstrate that metrical analysis can detect variations from symmetry in human skeletal material which then can be applied to interpretation of the conditions under which the population lived. The disruption to developmental stability of osseous structures, generating fluctuating asymmetries, may be attributed to pathological processes, genetic predisposition, congenital abnormalities, environmental influences, biomechanical stresses, or possibly a combination of these. Therefore, by creating an initial database of cranial and postcranial skeletal asymmetries, the existence and extent of asymmetries in a skeletal population can be used to detect deviations from the population norm and applied to differential diagnosis of individual departures from symmetry. This paper provides an example of this procedure.

Measurements and Methods

Of the 128 skeletal measurements being taken in a larger study, the current study selected 17 cranial and mandibular measurements as a test case to demonstrate the use of asymmetry studies. These measurements were applied to a small test sample of individuals from a rural parish in Hickelton (South Yorkshire) and from a leprosarium/almshouse in Chichester (West Sussex), two medieval skeletal populations held at the Biological Anthropology Research Centre (BARC), Department of Archaeological Sciences, University of Bradford. Twenty individuals were chosen for their completeness and lack of taphonomic changes that might affect measurement. The small size of the test sample is due to preservation and fragmentation limiting the overall number of obtainable measurements.

Seventeen cranial and mandibular measurements were taken for both the right and left sides (Table 1 and Figure 1). Each measurement was taken using either sliding calipers or spreading calipers, where appropriate. All measurements are based on standard cranial osteometric points and previously defined cranial measurements as described in Table 1 and Figure 1 (Howells 1973; White 1991; Moore-Jansen et al. 1994), except those used to obtain mastoid length, mastoid breadth, digastric groove length, and mandibular length (Table 1 and Figure 1). Here, mastoid length is defined as the distance from *porion* to *mastoidale*, as it was found that Howells' (1973) definition produced excessive measurement error. Mastoid breadth has similarly been adapted and is taken by placing the mastoid process between the calipers at the most posterior point and the most anterior point of its borders (Figure 1). Digastric groove length is defined as the maximum distance from the most anterior to the most posterior points of the digastric groove (Figure 1). Finally, mandibular length is taken using sliding calipers to measure from *condylion laterale* to *gnathion* (Figure 1).

The measurements were placed into a standard asymmetry equation: (R-L)/ ((R+L)/2). If the result was negative the trait was recorded as being left-sided. If the number was positive it was considered as favouring the right. A basic R-L formula was also used to show the degree of any deviation from symmetry. Once each individual was evaluated, these results were then compared with the standard deviation of the

measurements collected for the entire sample. Further, a standard intra-observer error was calculated on 11 complete skulls, taking measurements on both the left and the right sides to establish repeatability and accuracy.

Table 1: Cranial and Mandibular measurements (adapted from Moore-Jansen et al. 1994; White 1991; Howells 1973).

Measurement	Definition
Orbital breadth (ec-d)	The maximum internal distance from *dacryon* (d) to *ectoconchion* (ec), which can be found by bisecting the orbit into two halves with a straight edge keeping the line parallel with the super orbital border. This should be taken with sliding callipers.
Orbital height	The direct distance from the superior to the inferior orbital margins following a bisecting line thought the orbit perpendicular to orbital breadth. An internal measurement taken with sliding callipers.
Diagonal orbit breadth (nasion- or)(n-or)	The direct distance from *nasion* (n) to (or), using sliding callipers.
Frontomalare-nasion length (fmt-n)	The direct distance from *frontomalare* (fmt) to *nasion* (n), using sliding callipers.
Zygomatic height	The least distance from the most superior point on the lower margin of the orbit to the most superior point on the inferior border of the zygomatic, using sliding callipers.
Mastoid length (po-ms)	The direct distance from *porion* (po) to *mastoidale* (ms), using sliding callipers.
Mastoid breadth	Taken in the Frankfurt plane, the maximum distance is taken by placing the mastoid process between the callipers at the most posterior and the most anterior points along its borders.
Digastric groove length	The maximum distance from the most anterior to the most posterior points of the digastric groove. An internal measurement using sliding callipers.
Opisthion-porion length (o-po)	The direct distance from *opisthion* (o) to *porion* (po), using sliding callipers.
Basion-porion length (ba-po)	The direct distance from *basion* (ba) to *porion* (po), using sliding callipers.
Frontomalare-bregma length (fmt-b)	The direct distance from *frontomalare* (fmt) to *bregma* (b), using spreading callipers.
Bregma-porion length (b-po)	The direct distance from *bregma* (b) to *porion* (po), using spreading callipers.
Bregma-zygoorbitale length (b-zo)	The direct distance from *bregma* (b) to *zygoorbitale* (zo), using spreading callipers.
Mandibular length (cdl-gn)	The direct distance from *condylion laterale* (cdl) to *gnathion* (gn), using sliding callipers.
Max mandibular ramus height	The maximum distance from the most superior point on the condyle to the most inferior point on the inferior border of the corpus near the mandibular angle, using sliding callipers.
Max mandibular ramus breadth	The maximum distance from the most anterior point on the mandibular ramus at the coronoid process to the most posterior point on the condyle, using sliding callipers.
Min mandibular ramus breadth	The least breadth of the mandibular ramus, using sliding callipers.

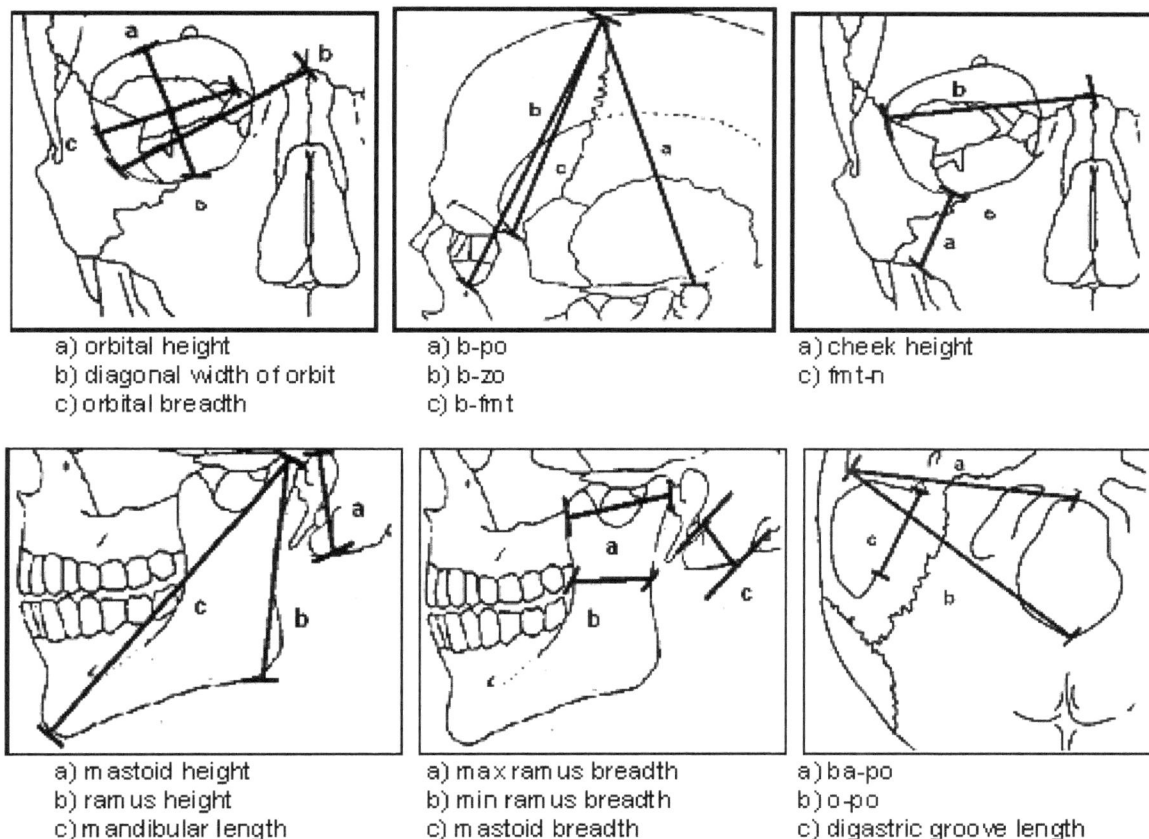

Figure 1: Measurements used. (Modified after Moore-Jansen et al. 1994)

Results

The measurements taken indicate that all the individuals exhibited at least some degree of cranial and mandibular asymmetry and that a right-sided asymmetry is the population norm. Mastoid length, mastoid breadth, *bregma-porion* length, orbital breadth, and mandibular ramus height measurements express the most asymmetry; while orbital height, diagonal orbital breadth, mandibular ramus breadth, and zygomatic height exhibit the least asymmetry (Table 2). The standard deviations of many of the measurements were found to be higher than those of other measurements, indicating fluctuating asymmetry in this population is variable. For instance, digastric groove length was the most variable within the population with a standard deviation of 3.0mm, followed by mastoid length with 2.8mm, *bregma-porion* length with 2.4mm, and *frontomalare-bregma* length with 2.3mm. The intra-observer error indicates that variation in each measurement was low with an error of +/-0.4mm or less.

Chichester 32, a young adult male, exhibited a noticeably exaggerated asymmetry as compared with the rest of the population (Table 2 and Figure 2).

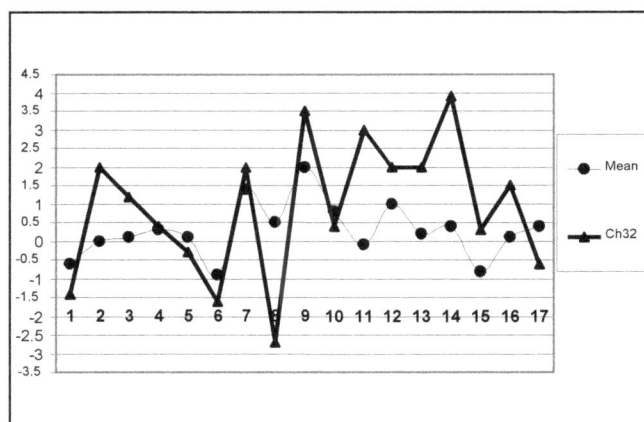

Figure 2: The differing asymmetry measurements of Chichester 32 compared with the population mean (most noticeable in orbital, frontal vault and mandibular asymmetries). Measurement number corresponds to those in Table 2.

Table 2: Descriptive Statistics for the population's 17 asymmetry measurements (mm). Negative numbers indicate the left side and positives the right. Ch 32 = Chichester skeleton 32.

Measurement number & summary	N	Min	Max	Mean	Std. Deviation	Ch 32	Observer error, *N*=22
1. Orbital breadth	12	-1.9	2.1	-0.6	1.1	-1.4	0.35
2. Orbital height	11	-1.3	2.0	0.0	1.2	2.0	0.24
3. Diagonal orbit breadth	9	-2.1	2.4	0.1	1.4	1.2	0.38
4. Ftm-n	17	-2.7	4.5	0.3	1.9	0.4	0.34
5. Zygomatic height	10	-0.6	1.3	0.1	0.6	-0.3	0.29
6. Mastoid length	15	-7.1	3.0	-0.9	2.8	-1.6	0.34
7. Mastoid breadth	13	-1.3	4.7	1.4	2.0	2.0	0.36
8. Digastric groove length	6	-2.7	5.7	0.5	3.0	-2.7	0.44
9. O-po	6	0.3	3.5	2.0	1.1	3.5	0.39
10. Ba-po	6	-0.1	2.0	0.8	0.9	0.4	0.37
11. Fmt-b	16	-5.0	3.0	-0.1	2.3	3	0.4
12. B-po	7	-2.0	5.0	1.0	2.4	2	0.36
13. B-zo	11	-4.0	3.0	0.2	2.1	2	0.4
14. Mandibular length	11	-2.1	4.0	0.4	1.6	3.9	0.31
15. Maximum ramus height	10	-3.8	1.8	-0.8	1.7	0.3	0.34
16. Maximum mandibular ramus breadth	10	-0.8	1.5	0.1	0.7	1.5	0.29
17. Minimum mandibular ramus breadth	12	-1.0	2.4	0.4	1.0	-0.6	0.25

Visual examination of the cranium revealed it to be malformed, as the orbits are asymmetrically shaped, the occipital abnormally flattened, and the left mastoid process under-developed. The extent of this malformation is more fully revealed through metric examination. For instance, the measurements of the orbits show the atrophied left side to be 1.4mm larger in breadth, a measurement that captures the unusual dimensions of the left orbit. The right orbit is 2.1mm larger in height and is positioned more than 1.2mm lower than that of the left side, which indicates the normal morphological position of the orbit (Figure 3).

The orbital measurements, breadth and diagonal breadth, deviate from the population mean as both are 1 standard deviation from the population mean, while orbital height is 2 standard deviations from the mean and in the opposite direction (Table 2). The right mastoid is broader by 2.0mm, while the left is 1.6mm longer with a 2.7mm longer digastric groove (Figure 4). These measurements indicate that it is the breadth of the mastoid process and not its length, nor that of the diagastric fossa, that relates to the atrophy noted. Both breadth and the length measurements differ from the mean by nearly 1mm side difference (Table 2). Furthermore, from the *opisthion-porion* measurement a noticeable deviation of the occipital to the left is seen (1 standard deviation from the mean), with the right measurement being 3.5mm longer than that of the left (Table 2 and Figure 4). The mandible is also malformed as the mandibular length is 3.9mm longer on the right (nearly 3 standard deviations from the mean), and the maximum ramus breadth is 1.5mm broader on the right (Table 2). These measurements indicate that the left side of the cranial vault and the left mandibular corpus is shorter and thus atrophied.

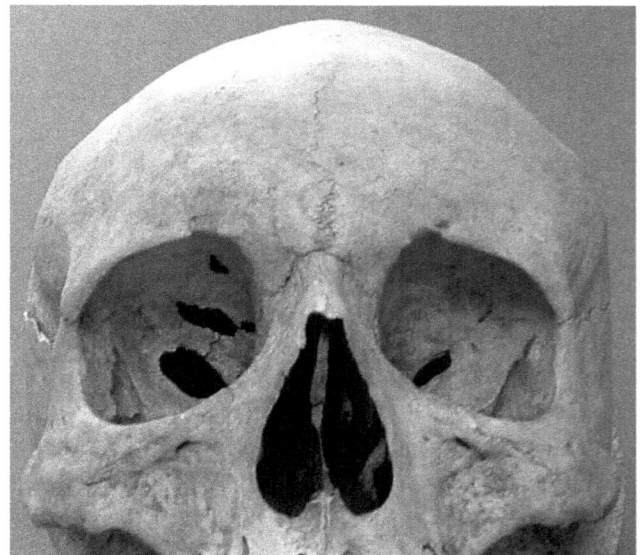

Figure 3: Atrophied left orbit of Chichester 32.

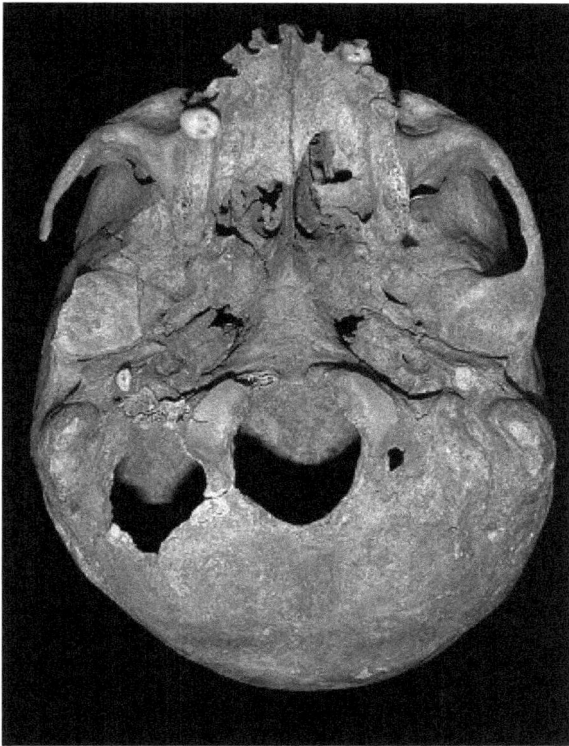

Figure 4: Chichester 32. Left deviation and right flattening of the occipital and enlarged right and under-developed left mastoid processes.

Discussion

The changes to the cranium of Chichester 32 seem to originate around the attachment of *M. sternocleidomastoideus*, which has been known to be involved in some congenital deformities. It has been suggested that within archaeological populations the type of asymmetrical development noted shares similarities with the clinical diagnosis of muscular torticollis (Knüsel 2002; Douglas 1991; Skinner et al. 1989), and it is likely that this may be the case with this individual. Chun-Yiu Cheng and co-workers state that, in recent populations, muscular torticollis is "one of the most common congenital problems of the musculoskeletal system in neonates and infants, with a reported incidence of 0.3% to 1.9%," (Chun-Yiu Cheng et al. 2000, 1237). Although the exact aetiology of muscular torticollis is still unknown, it seems to involve congenital damage to or failure of development of *M. sternocleidomastoideus* or of cranial nerve XI (accessory nerve) causing the head to be held in a laterally flexed position, which is associated with osseous changes such as flattening of the occipital the affected side, occipital bulging on the opposite side, torsion along the sagittal axis, asymmetrical mandible, and dropped orbit (Keller et al. 1986; Skinner et al. 1989; Douglas 1991; Chun-Yiu Cheng et al. 2000; Vaughn 2003). All of these are present in Chichester 32. The initial damage is postulated to occur during the strain of

labour when the fibers of *M. sternocleidomastoideus* tear during delivery or by the malposition of the infant *in utero*. Both are possible causes, as damage to this muscle has been observed both in infants from natural births and from caesarean sections (Skinner et al. 1989). Once *M. sternocleidomastoideus* is damaged, the mastoid process on the affected side is underdeveloped due to the lack of muscular development leaving the opposite side to be overdeveloped and unopposed such that the head tilts towards the unaffected side.

A differential diagnosis of these changes would be that they are due to biomechanical stress. It has been noted that *in utero* physical activities can also affect the skeletal growth of the foetus (Trenouth 1985; Carter et al. 1987; Hepper et al. 1991). Biomechanical stresses during growth and early life could also have contributed to fluctuating asymmetry. If this was the case, then an occupational origin might be inferred. However, the extreme asymmetry and atrophy of cranial superstructures such as the mastoid process suggest that the osseous changes are unlikely to have been created purely by biomechanical stress, but are most likely due to some congenital injury or condition.

Whatever the aetiology of the affliction, the skeletal changes could give insight into individual life experiences and into the population as a whole. On the population level, it can be said that a degree of developmental noise (i.e. low or minimal fluctuating asymmetry), is the norm. The population as a whole exhibited a degree of fluctuating asymmetry within the measurements, but they were not as drastic as seen in Chichester 32. The skeletal changes would most likely have given Chichester 32 a distinctive physical appearance and could have acted as a barrier to certain physical and social activities. Then inferences as to the social structure, health, genetic patterning, and environment and living conditions of both the individual and the population as a whole can be postulated. It is not only important to distinguish between the presence or absence of asymmetry in a measurement, but also to ascertain whether the asymmetry reflects that of the population, or is a divergence from the norm.

One of the main problems facing studies of fluctuating asymmetry is the possibility of intra-observer measurement error and taphonomic changes affecting the skeletal material being studied, such as twisting deformation due to the overburden of soil in burial. Although the taphonomic processes may compress the cranial vault, they cannot create the asymmetries found through measurement of bilateral structures. However, any observer error in measurement could either disguise or create false asymmetry readings within an individual. As has been shown, once the error estimate has been established and any effects of taphonomic processes noted, fluctuating asymmetry has the potential to add important information to osteological studies that would have otherwise been overlooked by observations based solely on non-metric examination of skeletal populations.

Acknowledgements

The authors would like to thank Holger Schutkowski, Darlene Weston, Anthea Boylston and Alan Ogden at the Biological Anthropology Research Centre at the University of Bradford for their help in developing the research protocol.

Literature Cited

Albert AM and Greene DL (1999) Bilateral Asymmetry in Skeletal Growth and Maturation as an Indicator of Environmental Stress. *American Journal of Physical Anthropology* 110: 341-349.

Carter DR, Orr TE, Fyrie DP, and Schurman, DJ (1987) Influences of Mechanical Stress on Prenatal and Postnatal Skeletal Development. *Clinical Orthopaedics and Related Research* 219: 237-250.

Chun-Yiu Cheng J, Metreweli C, Mui-Kwan Chen T, and Tang S-P (2000) Correlation of Ultrasonographic Imaging of Congenital Muscular Torticollis with Clinical Assessment in Infants. *Ultrasound in Medicine & Biology* 26 (8): 1237-1241.

Dittmar M (1998) Finger Ridge-Count Asymmetry and Diversity in Andean Indians and Interpopulation Comparisons. *American Journal of Physical Anthropology* 105: 377-393.

Douglas MT (1991) Wryneck in the ancient Hawaiians. *American Journal of Physical Anthropology* 84: 261-271.

Fields SJ, Spiers M, Hershkovitz I, and Livshits G (1995) Reliability of Relation Coefficients in the Estimation of Asymmetry. *American Journal of Physical Anthropology* 96: 83-87.

Hepper PG, Shahidullah S, and White R (1991) Handedness in the Human Fetus. *Neuropsychologia* 29 (11): 1107-1111.

Howells WW (1973) *Cranial Variation in Man: A Study by Multivariate of Patterns of Differences Among Recent Human Populations*. Peabody Museum of Archaeology and Ethnology Papers. Cambridge, MA: Harvard University Press.

Keller EE, Jackson, IT, Marsh WR, and Triplett WW (1986) Mandibular Asymmetry Associated with Congenital Muscular Tortocollis. Oral Surgery, Oral Medicine, Oral Pathology, *Oral Radiology and Endodontology* 61: 216-220.

Knüsel CJ (2002) More Circe than Cassandra: the Princess of Vix in ritualised social context. *Journal of European Archaeology* 5 (3): 275-308.

Larsen CS (1997) *Bioarchaeology: Interpreting Behavior from the Human Skeleton.* Cambridge University Press: Cambridge.

McManus C (2002) *Right Hand, Left Hand: The Origins of Asymmetry in Brains, Bodies, Atoms and Cultures.* London: Weidenfeld and Nicolson.

Moore-Jansen PM, Ousley SD, and Jantz RL (1994) *Data Collection Procedures for Forensic Skeletal Material.* Report of Investigations No. 48. Knoxville: University of Tennessee Press.

Palmer AR (1994) Fluctuating Asymmetry Analyses: A Primer. In TA Markow (ed.): *Developmental Instability: Its Origins and Evolutionary Implications.* Kluwer: Dordrech, the Netherlands; 335-364.

Skinner M, Barkley J, and Carlson RL (1989) Cranial Asymmetry and Muscular Torticollis in Prehistoric Northwest Coast Natives from British Columbia (Canada). *Journal of Paleopathology* 3 (1): 18-34.

Steele J and Mays S (1995) Handedness and Directional Asymmetry in the Long Bones of the Human Upper Limb. *International Journal of Osteoarchaeology* 5: 39-49.

Storm RA (2000) *Metrical Analysis of Asymmetry and Hand Preference in the Pectoral Girdle and Upper Arm as Observed in the Skeleton.* MSc Dissertation. Bradford: University of Bradford.

Trenouth MJ (1985) Asymmetry of the Human Skull During Fetal Growth. *Anatomical Record* 211 (2): 205-212.

White TD (1991) *Human Osteology.* San Diego, CA: Academic Press.

Van Valen L (1962) A Study of Fluctuating Asymmetry. *Evolution* 16: 125-42.

Vaughn BF (2003) Integrated Strategies for the Treatment of Spasmodic Torticollis. *Journal of Bodywork and Movement Therapies* 7 (3): 142-147.

The Adult Human Occipital Bone: Measurement Variance and Observer Error

Occiput: Measurement Variance and Observer Error

René Gapert* and Jason Last

Forensic Anthropology Study and Research Group
Department of Human Anatomy and Physiology, University College Dublin
Earlsfort Terrace, Dublin 2, Ireland.
*e-mail address for correspondence: rene.gapert@ucd.ie

Abstract

The adult human occipital bone offers opportunities to develop measurements that can aid in the identification of human remains, particularly as it tends to survive inhumation and physical insults more readily than many other bones of the skull. The occiput has a number of anatomical features, some of which have been evaluated for sex and ethnic differences including the occipital condyles and the foramen magnum. Using these features, ten measurements of the occipital region were chosen from past publications. In addition, the position of the hypoglossal canals offered an opportunity to develop two new measurements. Twenty skulls of unknown sex and ethnicity were obtained, their occipital regions examined, and a number of measurements performed. Twelve measurements were recorded to two decimal places using digital (Mitutoyo) sliding callipers. Parts A, B and C of this experiment examined intra-observer error, inter-observer error and variation between twenty skulls by using the coefficient of variation. This study aimed to define and evaluate measurements that may be used in identification of human cranial remains, and forms part of a wider study on sex differences of the condylar region of the human occipital bone. These initial results indicate that while all measurements have the potential to prove useful, the bicondylar breadth, the distance between the external hypoglossal canals, the length of the foramen magnum and the width of the foramen magnum are the most clearly defined, and may offer greatest potential in sex identification.

Keywords: Occipital, measurements, condyles, foramen magnum, hypoglossal, forensic anthropology, variation.

The human skull has been widely studied by anatomists and forensic physical anthropologists in order to define sex and ethnicity (Krogman 1978). Some of the earlier publications examined the whole skull for metric and observable traits (Parsons and Keene 1919) and used indices, such as the cranial index and facial index to establish sex differences. Researchers used different successful methods in identifying sex traits in the human skull by taking measurements of skulls from x-rays (Ceballos & Rentschler 1958), or recording measurements directly on the cranium and using discriminant function analysis to differentiate between the sexes (Giles & Elliot 1963).

The adult human occipital bone offers opportunities to develop measurements that can aid in the identification of human remains, particularly as it tends to survive inhumation and physical insults more readily than many other bones of the skull. It is therefore logical to examine the occipital region of the human skull for sex and ethnicity differences.

The occiput is found at the base of the cranium where it articulates with first cervical vertebra forming the atlanto-occipital joint. The cranial base has a number of anatomical features, some of which have been evaluated for sex and ethnicity differences including the occipital condyles and the foramen magnum. Some observers maintain that sexual differences in the occiput are better described than measured (Olivier 1975), while others believe that measurements and discriminant functions are useful to a certain degree (Holland 1986). Here, ten measurements of the occipital region were chosen from past publications (Routal et al. 1984; Holland 1986). In addition, the position of the hypoglossal canals offered an opportunity to develop two new measurements.

In taking any measurements, observer and random errors occur. Further errors occur when the points between which distances are measured are not clearly defined. This study aims to establish, through analysis of variance, the measurements that yield consistent results. This phase of the study must precede any examination of ethnicity and sex differences to ensure the integrity of the techniques used.

Materials and Methods

Twenty skulls of unknown sex and ethnicity were obtained from anatomical supply companies and the craniology collection in University College Dublin. The occipital regions were examined, and a number of measurements performed. Twelve measurements were recorded to two decimal places using digital (Mitutoyo) sliding calipers (Table 1).

Table 1. Description of measurements.

Code	Measurement
MLC	Maximum length of occipital condyle
MWC	Maximum width of occipital condyle
MnD	Minimum distance between the medial borders of the condyles
MxID	Maximum distance between the medial borders of the condyles
BCB	Bicondylar breadth
LFM	Length of the foramen magnum
WFM	Width of the foramen magnum
FMC	Circumference of the foramen magnum
LBP	Length of basilar process
DF	Distance between the postcondyloid foramina
HCH	Height of the occipital condyles
EHC	Distance between the external openings of the hypoglossal canals

Ten measurements were chosen from past publications (Routal et al. 1984; Holland 1986): the maximum length of the occipital condyle (MLC) taken from the most anterior point to the most posterior point of the articular surface, the maximum width of occipital condyle (MWC) taken at the most lateral point to the most medial point of the articular surface, the minimum distance between the medial borders of the condyles (MnD) taken at the articular surface, the maximum distance between the medial borders of the condyles (MxID) taken at the articular surface, the bicondylar breadth (BCB) taken between the most lateral points of the condylar articular surfaces, the length of the foramen magnum (LFM) using the maximum internal length, the width of the foramen magnum (WFM) using the maximum internal width, the circumference of the foramen magnum (FMC) using a strip of graph paper which is then pressed against the internal borders of the foramen magnum, marked and then measured with digital sliding calipers, the length of the basilar process (LBP) taken from the most anterior point on the internal border of the foramen magnum in the midline to the midpoint of the suture of the spheno-occipital synchondrosis, and the distance between postcondyloid foramina (DF) taken by measuring from the midpoint of each foramina.

The two new measurements developed by the authors were the height of the occipital condyles (HCH) taken from the floor of the internal hypoglossal canal to the maximum convexity of the condylar articular surface, and the distance between the external openings of the hypoglossal canals (EHC) taken from the medial walls of the external hypoglossal canals.

For analysis, the coefficient of variation (CV) was used. This is a measure of relative dispersion and generally expressed as a percentage.

Part A

A single set of twelve measurements was recorded on each of the twenty skulls by one observer. The CV was calculated for each measurement to serve as an index demonstrating the amount of variation between skulls.

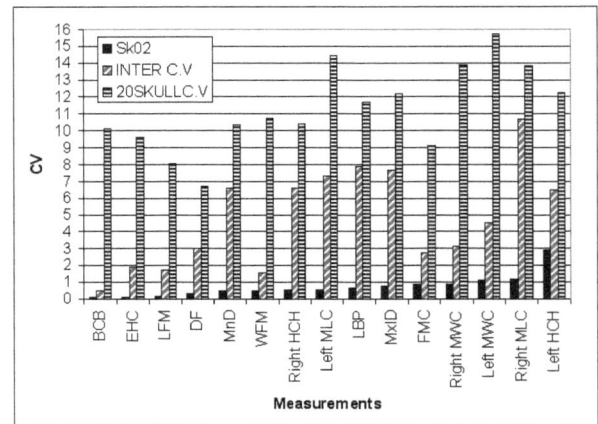

Figure 1. Skull SK02 intra-observer coefficient of variation (CV) compared to inter-observer CV and variation between 20 skulls for all twelve measurements. 20SKULLC.V. refers to Part A, INTER C.V. refers to Part B and Sk02 refers to Part C.

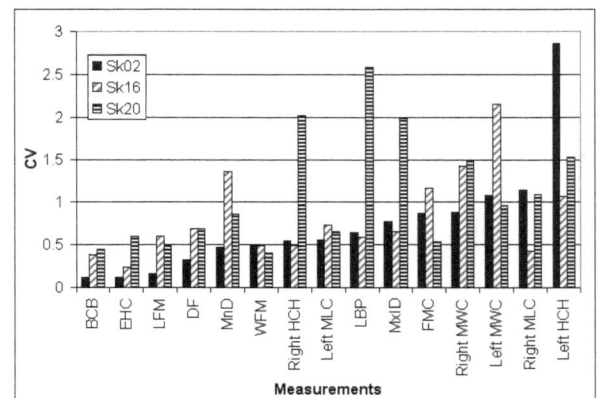

Figure 2: Comparison of intra-observer coefficients of variation (CVs) between skulls SK02, SK16 and SK20. The bicondylar breadth (BCB), external hypoglossal canal distance (EHC), the width of the foramen magnum (WFM) and the length of the foramen magnum (LFM) have consistently low CVs.

Part B

This part consisted of using the set of twelve measurements on three skulls (SK2, SK16 and SK20), measuring each skull twenty times in order to record intra-observer error (Figs. 1, 2). These were performed by the same observer as in Part A. Each of the three skulls had been measured on different days. On each day, a set of twelve measurements was taken, and the process repeated twenty times. Once more, the coefficient of variation was calculated. However, the CV here serves as an indicator of error in the measurement process. This error is a combination of intra-observer error, random error and error due to the ambiguity of the landmarks that guide each measurement.

Part C
Inter-observer error was examined in Part C of the experiment by asking ten different observers to take the twelve measurements on one skull (SK02) (Fig 1).

The observers were lecturers and postgraduate tutors of the Department of Human Anatomy and Physiology at University College Dublin. All observers were also familiar with the occiput and but none had previous knowledge of the measurements in Table 1. Each observer was given a list of measurements with instructions. The list had been prepared by the observer for Part A and B. This was accompanied by a practical demonstration performed by the authors. The CV in this part indicates the error between observers, in addition to error inherent in the feature measured.

Results

Part A allowed the calculation of the mean and range of values for each measurement from a group of 20 different skulls. The CVs for the measurements varied between 6.72 and 15.73. These figures indicate the percentage standard deviation from the mean. The LBP could not be recorded in 75% of skulls, nor the DF in 60%. The reasons for this were the obliteration of the spheno-occipital synchondrosis and the lack of patent postcondyloid foramina in some skulls.

In Part B, where three skulls were measured, intra-observer CV's for skulls SK2, SK16 and SK20 ranged from 0.11 to 2.85, 0.24 to 2.15 and 0.41 to 2.58 respectively (see Fig. 2). The closer the observer variations are to the variation found between the twenty different skulls in Part A, the less likely the measurement in question is to be of use for future assessment as to applicability for sex determination. The most favourable measurements by this analysis were BCB, EHC, WFM and LFM.

In Part C, which examined inter-observer error, the CVs for all twelve measurements demonstrate that the most precise measurements are BCB, EHC, WFM and LFM (Fig. 1).

Discussion

The adult human occipital bone tends to survive inhumation and physical insults more readily than other

bones of the cranium. It is therefore logical to examine the occipital region of the human skull for sex and ethnicity differences. Some observers maintain that sexual differences in the occiput are better described than measured (Olivier 1975), while others believe that measurements and discriminant functions are useful to a certain degree (Holland 1986). The condylar and foramen magnum region were examined in this study. Ten measurements were utilised from past publications (Routal et al. 1984; Holland 1986), and two additional new measurements were devised (Table 1). It was noted by other researchers that Holland's measurements were difficult to replicate with precision and that the measurements of the foramen magnum were the most reliable. Also, significant sex and ethnicity variation was found to be present in the condylar region (Westcott & Moore-Jansen, 2001).

This study indicates that certain measurements are more clearly defined than others, and therefore some may be more accurately reproduced by a multitude of observers. Some descriptions of measurements lack definition due to the ambiguity of the feature measured. The maximum length and width of the foramen magnum as well as the distance between the external openings of the hypoglossal canals seem to be straightforward features. The length and width of the articular surfaces of the occipital condyles lack definition in comparison. The problem with these structures is that sometimes the surface margins, and especially the posterior border of the occipital condyles, are indistinguishable from the surrounding ex-occipital structures. Other contributing factors that make definition of the margins difficult include erosion of and damage to the articular surfaces, including by the repetitive use of sliding calipers, as the points of the instrument may chip tiny bone pieces off the articular surface border. The reason for this study is to test some of the established methods for accuracy and consistency, and therefore the sex of the skulls in the sample was of no consequence to this study. The number of skulls chosen for this project was based on previous research (Westcott & Moore-Jansen 2001). New measurements have been added and form part of a larger research project on sexual dimorphism in the human occipital bone at University College Dublin. Methods for sex identification in the foramen magnum area developed by Teixeria (1982), Routal et al (1984) and Holland (1986) showed limitations. Teixeria's (1982) methodology had been examined by Günay and Altinkök (2000), while Holland's (1986) method had been tested by Westcott and Moore-Jansen (2001) and was found to contain inconsistencies in measurement definition. Westcott and Moore-Jansen concluded that Holland's models could not estimate sex or ethnicity with more than 76% accuracy. The results in Part A of this study confirm past findings (Williams 1987; Westcott & Moore-Jansen 2001) that firstly, the length of the basilar process cannot be recorded due to suture obliteration of the spheno-occipital synchondrosis in many cases and secondly, the distance between the openings of the postcondyloid foramina cannot be recorded due to absence of one or both of the foramina in many cases.

The results of Part A of this study show that there is substantial variation in the features of the occipital region between individual skulls. Such differences could be due to sex, ethnicity, pathology or other genetic and environmental factors. Part B and C suggest that some measurements are easier and more accurately recorded than others. Some factors, such as well-defined features and the demonstration of how to take the measurements to a multitude of observers, play a role in deciding which measurements are more favourable. The findings also support Westcott and Moore-Jansen's (2001) statement that some measurements put forward by Holland (1986) are difficult to replicate precisely. However, the results obtained also indicate that morphological differences exist in the occipital region, and these may offer opportunities to identify sex in the cranial base by metrical analysis.

Conclusions

This study aimed to define and evaluate measurements that may be used in identification of human cranial remains, and forms part of a wider study on sexual differences of the condylar region of the human occipital bone. These initial results indicate that while all measurements have the potential to prove useful, the BCB, EHC LFM and WFM are the most clearly defined, and may offer greatest potential in sex identification.

Acknowledgements

We would like to thank Sue Black, University of Dundee and Director of CIFA, John Bannigan, Head of Department of Human Anatomy and Physiology, University College Dublin, Raj Ettarh, Jennifer Thompson, Eoin Hipwell, Edward Dervan, Aine Dowling, Marie Meskell and Anne Marie O'Donnell, all from University College Dublin. Ulrich Schmidt, Institute for Forensic Medicine, Heinrich-Heine University, Düsseldorf, Germany.

Literature Cited

Ceballos JL and Rentschler EH (1958) Roentgen diagnosis of sex based on adult skull characteristics. *Radiology* 70: 55-61.

Giles E and Elliot O (1963) Sex determination by discriminant function analysis of crania. *American Journal of Physical Anthropology* 21: 53-68.

Günay Y and Altinkök M (2000) The value of the size of foramen magnum in sex determination. Short Report. *Journal of Clinical Forensic Medicine* 7: 147-149.

Holland TD (1986) Sex determination of fragmentary crania by analysis of the cranial base. *American Journal of Physical Anthropology* 70: 203-208.

Krogman WM (1978) *The Human Skeleton in Forensic Medicine,* 3rd edition. Springfield: Charles C. Thomas.

Olivier G (1975) Biometry of the human occipital bone. *Journal of Anatomy* 120: 507-518.

Parsons FG and Keene L (1919) Sexual differences in the skull. *Journal of Anatomy* 54: 58-65.

Routal et al (1984) Metrical studies with sexual dimorphism in foramen magnum of human crania. *Journal of the Anatomical Society of India* 33: 85-89.

Teixeria WRG (1982) Sex identification utilizing the size of the foramen magnum. *American Journal of Forensic Medicine and Pathology* 3: 203-206.

Westcott DJ and Moore-Jansen PH (2001) Metric variation in the human occipital bone: forensic anthropological applications. *Journal of Forensic Sciences* 46: 1159-1163.

Williams MM (1987) *Sex determination of fragmentary crania by analysis of the cranial base: applications for the study of an Arikara skeletal sample.* Thesis. University of Tennessee.

Estimating Age at Death from the Pubic Symphysis: Past, Present and Future.

Pubic Symphysis Age at Death

Rebecca Gowland[1]* and Andrew T. Chamberlain[2]

[1] St John's College, University of Cambridge
Cambridge, CB2 1TP.

[2] Department of Archaeology, University of Sheffield
Northgate House, West Street, Sheffield, S1 4ET.

* e-mail address for correspondence: rlg31@cam.ac.uk

Abstract

The ability of biological anthropologists to determine accurately the mortality profiles of skeletal samples has been under serious doubt over the last two decades. As one of the primary methods of age estimation, the pubic symphysis has frequently been at the heart of attempts to produce accurate and reliable estimations of skeletal age at death. This study provides a review of pubic symphyseal ageing methods over the last century and identifies some of the problems associated with current techniques. Recent publications on skeletal age estimation have explored the use of Bayesian and maximum likelihood methods. Here we set out how Bayesian statistics can be used in a straightforward manner to estimate the mortality distribution of archaeological skeletal populations with widely varying mortality profiles, using the Suchey-Brooks system of pubic symphyseal stages. The Bayesian method is also tested on a known age skeletal sample. This paper provides some encouraging results and demonstrates that, by incorporating Bayesian statistics into a pubic symphyseal ageing method, archaeologists can in fact obtain valid approximations of the mortality distributions of past populations.

Keywords: Pubic Symphysis, Age Estimation, Bayesian, Demography, Skeletal Populations

Introduction

Estimation of the chronological age of the adult skeleton from the morphological appearance of the bones and teeth is an important but challenging problem in forensic anthropology and palaeodemography. The subchondral surface of the pubic symphysis is particularly suitable for adult age estimation because it exhibits clearly defined changes that reflect both skeletal development and senescence, thus the changes that occur at the pubic symphysis span the full range of adult life. Todd (1920, 1921a, 1921b) was the first to map the changing state of the pubic symphysis, observing the surface texture and topography of the symphyseal face, dorsal and ventral surfaces (including the formation of the ventral rampart), and superior and inferior surfaces. Since the pioneering work of Todd, the pubic symphysis method has undergone numerous tests, revisions and new approaches (Suchey et al. 1986) and it continues to be the subject of intensive anthropological investigation (Pasquier et al. 1999; Hoppa 2000; Schmitt et al. 2002; Hoppa & Sitchon 2003; Schmitt 2004). As a result the pubic symphysis has undergone more analysis and testing than any other skeletal criterion of age estimation.

One of the fundamental problems with the pubic symphysis as an age indicator is the variability exhibited in both the timing and nature of the changes between individuals. This variability becomes particularly marked over the age of approximately 35 years, once the ventral rampart has fused and all changes become degenerative (Saunders et al. 1992; Meindl & Russell 1998). This chronological variability in skeletal degeneration between individuals and the extent to which the morphological changes may be influenced by physical stress are factors that confound all skeletal ageing methods. As discussed previously, while Todd (1920) argued that the pubic symphysis was affected by lifestyle and disease, he did not believe that childbirth had any impact on the changes observed (Todd 1921b: 40). However, for some time it has also been acknowledged that females exhibit more variability than males, both in terms of the nature of the changes occurring and their chronology (Stewart 1957; Gilbert 1973; Suchey 1979). This is partly the result of obstetric factors, although mechanical stress may also contribute to variation at the pubic symphysis. Klepinger et al.'s (1992) study of a forensic sample found that severe physical trauma, or lack of normal physical activity through disability, affected the sequence of morphological changes (Klepinger et al. 1992: 768).

This paper provides a review of pubic symphyseal ageing

methods and addresses current debates concerning skeletal age estimation. We identify some of the problems with current techniques, collate known age pubic symphysis data, and apply a Bayesian statistical method to archaeological skeletal populations to examine whether reliable demographic profiles are attainable.

Pubic Symphyseal Ageing

Past

Todd (1920) initially based his method on a collection of 306 white male skeletons of known age at death. He identified nine areas of the symphyseal face whose changing state he mapped through ten distinct phases, selecting 'typical' examples to represent each morphological phase. Todd (1920: 327) noted that a degree of inter-individual variability existed, particularly with respect to those individuals exhibiting signs of disease. However, in a subsequent study of female pubic bones Todd (1921b: 40) argued that there were no discernible differences relating to parturition in females, stating 'I do not believe that pregnancy and child-birth leave any permanent stamp on the skeleton'. Todd's method remained unchallenged until a study by Brooks (1955) found that it produced inaccurate results and demonstrated a tendency to overage in the third decade. In an attempt to improve on Todd's original method, Brooks (1955) introduced a number of modifications to his ten-stage system. Casts were also developed in order to more clearly display the 'typical' features of each stage and diminish inter-observer variability.

A more drastic overhaul of the pubic symphyseal method was then undertaken by McKern and Stewart (1957), based on a new known-age skeletal reference series. They argued that Todd's system oversimplified the changes occurring in the pubic symphyseal face and did not allow sufficiently for individual variability. McKern and Stewart (1957) stated that certain components of the symphyseal face changed independently and must be examined and recorded accordingly. McKern and Stewart devised a three-component system, whereby the metamorphosis of three features of the symphyseal face (the dorsal demi-face, the ventral demi-face, and the symphyseal rim) were observed and recorded separately. Each component was divided into five developmental stages and scored accordingly; the sum of these scores was then converted into an age estimate.

A similar component system was devised by Gilbert and McKern (1973) for females. They observed that the female symphyseal face underwent accelerated rates of morphological change in certain areas, most notably the dorsal surface, causing inaccuracies in age estimates (Gilbert 1973). This factor was also noted by Stewart (1957) who argued, contrary to Todd (1921), that this was likely to be the result of trauma associated with childbirth. Although these component systems were initially believed to improve age estimates by allowing greater objectivity (Hanihara & Suzuki 1978), blind tests of the component methods and comparisons with other pubic symphysis methods have demonstrated that they were in fact prone to greater inaccuracies than traditional methods. Gilbert and McKern's (1973) female standard was tested by Suchey (1979) who found that only 51% of estimates were within fifteen years of documented age. Suchey (1979) believed that this inaccuracy was not entirely the result of the variability of female symphyses, but rather with faults inherent to the Gilbert and McKern system (e.g. a high degree of inter-observer error associated with difficulties identifying the stages described).

Meindl et al. (1985) and Meindl and Lovejoy (1989) also found component systems to be less 'biologically sensitive'; instead they found Todd's (1920) original method with the modifications suggested by Brooks (1955) to be more accurate. They produced a system that recognised five major biological phases for the pubic symphysis (Meindl et al. 1985). This system was criticised on the grounds that some of the ages assigned to their reference series (the Hamann Todd collection) were questionable (Suchey et al. 1986; Katz & Suchey 1989), a criticism that was later refuted by Meindl et al. (1990).

Nemeskéri et al.'s (1960) pubic symphyseal method (which later formed part of the complex method of Acsádi & Nemeskéri 1970) also recognised only five separate developmental phases. However, these authors were criticised by Brooks and Suchey (1990) for concentrating solely on early and late developmental features and indeed this is very evident when one compares their stages to those of other published methods. The 'Complex Method' was tested by Molleson and Cox (1993) on the Spitalfields known age skeletal collection and was found to underage older individuals and overage younger individuals quite substantially.

These studies (together with others not cited here) testify to a long-standing interest in age estimation using the pubic symphysis, both amongst forensic anthropologists and bioarchaeologists. Despite the problems identified above, the pubic symphysis has proved to be of sufficient utility to warrant its continuing use as one of a range of methods for estimation of age from the skeleton.

Present

The 'Suchey-Brooks' system (Brooks & Suchey 1990) is the method most commonly used in the UK at present. Using pubic bones from 739 males and 273 females from post-mortem cases, Suchey and Brooks devised a system comprising six phases each for males and females and these were groupings of Todd's (1920) original ten

Table 1: Age ranges associated with each pubic symphyseal phase for males & females (after Brooks & Suchey 1990).

Phase	Female (n=273)			Male (n=739)		
	Mean	*S.D.*	*95% range*	*Mean*	*S.D.*	*95% range*
I	19.4	2.6	15-24	18.5	2.1	15-23
II	25.0	4.9	19-40	23.4	3.6	19-34
III	30.7	8.1	21-53	28.7	6.5	21-46
IV	38.2	10.9	26-70	35.2	9.4	23-57
V	48.1	14.6	25-83	45.6	10.4	27-66
VI	60.0	12.4	42-87	61.2	12.2	34-86

phases. Exemplar casts are available of each phase, greatly assisting the consistent application of the method. In an independent test, this method has been found to outperform other pubic symphyseal ageing techniques (Klepinger et al. 1992). As with the majority of ageing methods, in blind tests, younger adults were aged with a much greater degree of accuracy than older adults.

A problem encountered when using the Suchey-Brooks method, however, is the broad error ranges provided (Table 1). These error ranges highlight the problem of variability discussed previously and have led workers to question the usefulness of the pubic symphysis ageing method. Work within the field of palaeodemography has seriously questioned the ability of skeletal age indicators to provide reliable demographic profiles of past populations (e.g. Bocquet-Appel & Masset 1982, 1985). This in part stems from the problem of skeletal variability, resulting in a poor correlation between age indicators and chronological age. This poor correlation has been shown to result in a statistical bias towards the age structure of the reference series on which the method is based. Hence, the age structures of our target archaeological sample become influenced by the age structure of a skeletal series entirely unconnected with the target sample.

Furthermore, Hoppa (2000) has recently demonstrated that one of the most fundamental assumptions of human skeletal ageing, that the chronology of age indicators in modern skeletal reference populations will be similar to past populations, is flawed. Hoppa recorded the pubic symphysis phases of the reference series used in Brooks and Suchey's method and compared these to two other reference series: one forensic and one recent archaeological. Hoppa (2000: 188) found that 'the rate of early development and later degeneration between the three relatively contemporaneous series is different, and significantly so for females.' This refutation of the uniformitarian stance necessarily taken by physical anthropologists is very important as it contributes yet another confounding element of variation. So the question remains: can we obtain useful demographic profiles from archaeological samples of human skeletal remains?

Future

Recent publications on skeletal age estimation have explored the use of Bayesian and maximum likelihood methods (e.g. Konigsberg & Frankenberg 1992; Chamberlain 2000; Gowland & Chamberlain 2002; Hoppa & Vaupel 2002). Bayesian data analysis allows us to make inferences from data using probability models for observable quantities (known age data) and for quantities that are unknown (archaeological data), but we wish to learn about (Gelman et al. 1995: 3). The fundamental necessity of Bayesian inference in palaeodemographic age-at-death estimation of skeletal populations has been emphasised by Hoppa and Vaupel (2002: 2), although some biological anthropologists have expressed reservations about the utility of Bayesian techniques (for example, Bocquet-Appel & Masset 1996; Mays 2003).

A method for ageing individuals using 'transition analysis' has recently been published by Boldsen and colleagues (2002). This method employs the principles of Bayesian inference for the estimation of skeletal age based on multiple age indicators (including the pubic symphysis, auricular surface and cranial suture closure). For the pubic symphysis, Boldsen et al. (2002) have revised the McKern and Stewart component method and they provide a statistical argument for component rather than 'type' methods. Their method is reported to perform well in independent tests, and it may prove to be suitable for use by academic and professional osteoarchaeologists when the computer programs required become more widely available.

Here we set out how Bayesian statistics can be used in a straightforward manner to estimate the mortality distribution of archaeological skeletal populations with widely varying mortality profiles, using the Suchey-Brooks system of pubic symphyseal stages (Brooks & Suchey 1990). Our aims are to determine whether the pubic symphysis can be used to generate plausible demographic profiles from archaeological samples.

Table 2: Archaeological samples examined in this study

Site	Site Period	Site Type	No. of Adults	No. of Adults with Pubic Symphyses
Lankhills, Hampshire	Late Roman	Attritional Cemetery	307	67 (21.8%)
Cassington, Oxfordshire	Late Roman	Unknown	53	18 (33.9%)
Abingdon, Oxfordshire	Early Saxon	Attritional Cemetery	79	29 (36.7%)
Blackgate, Newcastle	Medieval	Attritional Cemetery	469	84 (18.9%)
Royal Mint, London	Medieval	Plague Cemetery	363	70 (19.3%)

(NB the number of adults examined at the Royal Mint site was a sample of a total number of 420 individuals over the age of 15 years from the site (Margerison & Knüsel 2002: 137-138).

Materials and Methods

From Table 2 it is apparent that the sites examined in this study vary considerably in terms of chronological period and size and type of skeletal assemblage. We deliberately set out to test our methods on sites that are likely to have very different age-at-death profiles. From Table 2 it is also apparent that the pubic symphysis tends not to be well preserved in archaeological remains. This is because the pubic symphysis is fragile, especially in archaeological skeletons, as it contains a high proportion of cancellous bone (which is more prone to degradation than compact bone), and its exposed position when the skeleton is supine means that it is vulnerable to mechanical disturbance. The small proportion of pubic symphyses preserved means that we are attempting to examine the demography of a site from only a small sample of the total number of adult skeletons from what is probably an incompletely excavated cemetery. Even if a cemetery is entirely excavated, the individuals buried will not represent the entire population, and those skeletons with an intact pubic symphysis are a further sub-sample of the available material.

All of the pubic symphyses from these cemetery sites were recorded using the stages defined by Brooks and Suchey (1990) and with the aid of the casts depicting typical appearances of the stages in males and females. The sex of the skeletons was estimated using standard criteria prior to assessing the pubic symphysis stage. It was noted that many female pubic symphyses displayed atypical features, and often did not correspond to the descriptions or casts produced by Brooks and Suchey (1990). The female pubic symphyses from several sites (in particular from Lankhills) were also extremely gracile and this led to further difficulties in estimating age phase. By contrast, the male pubic symphyses displayed much more regularity in age related changes and exhibited far fewer ambiguous cases. A demographic profile of each of these cemeteries has been produced using the Bayesian method outlined below.

Bayesian Method

In order to produce a Bayesian age profile, a large series of pubic symphyses from known age skeletons must be recorded in order to construct a probability model so that the probability of age given pubic symphysis stage can be determined. The pubic symphyses of a total of 377 individuals were recorded from skeletons of known age of death from the Coimbra Identified Skeletal Collection, Portugal and the Spitalfields skeletal collection, London, using the Brooks and Suchey (1990) method. Two known-age skeletal series were recorded to ensure an adequate dataset and in the light of evidence that there is variation among reference series in the rate of progression of changes at the pubic symphysis (Hoppa 2000). In order to eliminate inter-observer error, the first author recorded all of these data, together with those obtained from the archaeological skeletal populations.

The males and females were assigned to pubic symphysis stages using the descriptions provided by Brooks and Suchey (1990) and the information in the instructional materials accompanying the pubic symphysis casts. The co-distribution of age and symphysis stage in the combined Coimbra and Spitalfields reference series was then used as a source of likelihoods (the probability of possessing a particular skeletal indicator stage given known age). It was found that, although females tended to show a greater variability in the stages that they expressed, there was no substantial difference between the sexes allowing us to pool the male and female data to produce a smoother probability distribution (for any given age category, males and females on average differed by less than half of one indicator stage). The likelihoods based on this pooled distribution were therefore used to provide probabilities of age given each skeletal indicator stage (Table 3) by using a Bayesian calculation and incorporating model prior probabilities:

$$p(A_i | I_j) = \frac{p(I_j | A_i) \times p(A_i)}{p(I_j)}$$

Table 3: The posterior probabilities of age given pubic symphysis stage when assuming an attritional model prior.

Age	Pubic Symphysis Stage					
	1	2	3	4	5	6
16-24	0.910	0.393	0.059			
25-34	0.090	0.321	0.509	0.196	0.046	0.013
35-44		0.135	0.178	0.291	0.135	0.041
45-54		0.097	0.122	0.225	0.158	0.112
55-64			0.038	0.155	0.276	0.247
65-74			0.093	0.102	0.246	0.323
75-99				0.030	0.139	0.264

In the above equation, $p(A_i|I_j)$, represents the probability of being in age category i given the particular indicator state j and is referred to as the *posterior probability*, as it represents opinion that is revised in reference to the datum, after observing the indicator state represented by I_j. The probability of possessing a particular indicator state given age, shown in the equation as $pI_j|A_i$), is calculated from the reference series and is referred to as the *likelihood*, as it is the conditional probability of possessing indicator state j given a particular age category i. The overall probability of possessing a particular indicator state is represented by $p(I_j)$, calculated as the sum of [$p(I_j|A_i) \times p(A_i)$] over all categories of A. The term $p(A_i)$ is referred to as the *prior probability* because it represents an opinion of the probability of being in A_i before any data has been observed (Phillips, 1973). By using a prior probability we are explicitly stating our prior beliefs concerning the data.

Choice of Prior

In the use of Bayesian statistics the choice of prior $p(A_i)$ is important as it will have some impact upon the results, particularly so for those skeletal indicators that have a poor correlation with chronological age (Aykroyd et al., 1997). There are several approaches that one can adopt when determining the value of $p(A_i)$. The 'Rostock Manifesto', as outlined by Hoppa and Vaupel (2002) recommends that this value should be derived from the archaeological data itself, by modelling the age distribution most likely to have generated the distribution of skeletal indicators in the archaeological sample. However, this requires that the archaeological sample be of a sufficient size and of unbiased composition in order to provide useful estimates of $p(A_i)$ (Boldsen et al., 2002). Another approach is to assume that the value of $p(A_i)$ is equal for all age categories (i.e. a uniform prior probability). However, because population mortality profiles rarely have equal proportions of deaths across all age categories this would not normally provide the most appropriate values.

The approach adopted here is to use prior probabilities based on model life tables. The reason for this is that

patterns of human mortality generally demonstrate a high degree of uniformity across populations (Paine 2000: 181). When producing the demographic profile of a 'normal' cemetery (i.e. one used for the burial of natural deaths over a long time period) we would expect natural attritional mortality: characterized by a high number of infant deaths, low numbers of adolescent deaths, and a gradual increase in mortality throughout adulthood (Paine 2000: 181). The data used for the model priors in this study were obtained from Coale and Demeny's Level 5 model west life tables for stable populations with zero rate of growth (Coale & Demeny 1983). For modelling attritional mortality we used the age distribution of deaths in the model life tables, and for modelling catastrophic mortality we used the age distributions of the living model life table populations. We argue that this approach is more satisfactory than that outlined by Hoppa and Vaupel (2002), because it is less likely to incorporate preservational and sampling biases into the age estimation. Although an attritional mortality pattern is not expected from *all* of the archaeological sites examined in this study, we treat the attritional pattern as the default prior and substitute the catastrophic prior only when it is warranted by the resulting age distribution.

Results and Discussion

When we examine the age profiles generated by the Bayesian ageing methods it is apparent that there are primarily two different types of mortality distribution represented amongst the archaeological samples. Three of the sites (Cassington, Lankhills and Blackgate) exhibited a mortality distribution that is similar to the attritional mortality model taken from Coale and Demeny's model west 5 population (Fig. 1). Despite the very small proportion of pubic symphyses surviving in a recordable state from the archaeological populations, we are still able to derive an age-at-death distribution that approximates that expected from a cemetery of this type.

Two of the sites in the dataset, Abingdon and the Royal Mint, exhibited mortality distributions that appeared not to be attritional but are compatible with that expected from a catastrophic mortality pattern (Fig. 2).

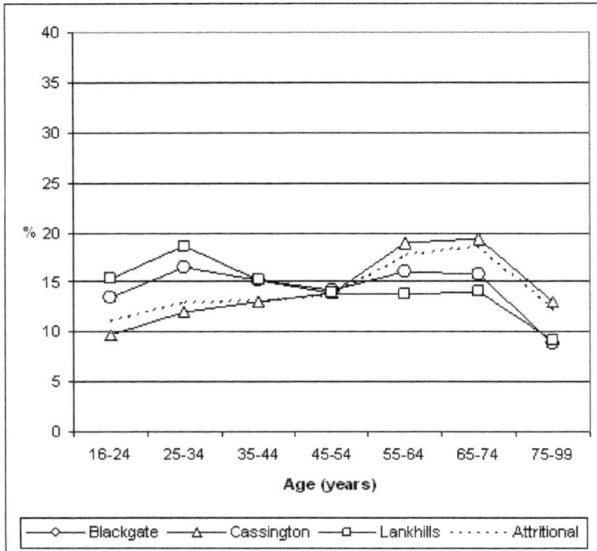

Figure 1: The sites exhibiting an attritional mortality distribution when age is estimated from the pubic symphyses using an attritional prior.

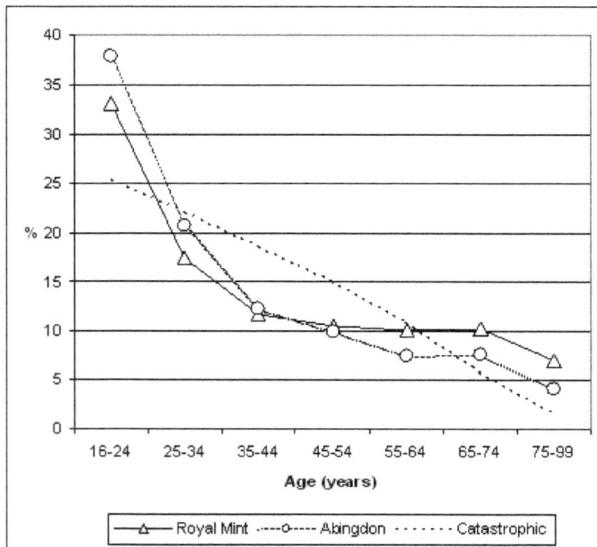

Figure 2: The sites exhibiting a catastrophic mortality distribution when age is estimated from the pubic symphyses using an attritional prior.

Catastrophic mortality refers to a short-term mortality crisis in which a high risk of death applies to all age categories. A catastrophic mortality profile should mimic the age structure of the living population because all individuals have an approximately equal probability of dying irrespective of age or sex (Keckler 1997). The skeletal sample from the Royal Mint site is believed to contain some of the victims of the Black Death plague (Grainger and Hawkins 1988), an epidemic that is likely

to have resulted in a catastrophic mortality pattern. Although no detailed documents relating to Black Death plague mortality exist, Gowland and Chamberlain (in press) found that parish records available for later plague episodes in Europe produced catastrophic mortality patterns that were very similar to that of the Royal Mint site.

These results are encouraging as they demonstrate that even though an attritional prior probability was used, alternative mortality profiles can clearly be distinguished in the archaeological mortality profiles. Given that the Abingdon and Royal Mint mortality distributions resembled the catastrophic profile we recalculated the age distributions for these cemeteries using a catastrophic prior probability (i.e. that of the living population). The results do not differ greatly from those obtained with an attritional prior, but they provide a slightly better match with the model catastrophic profile (Fig. 3). This indicates that the age distributions of the archaeological populations are not too greatly influenced by choosing between an attritional and a catastrophic prior.

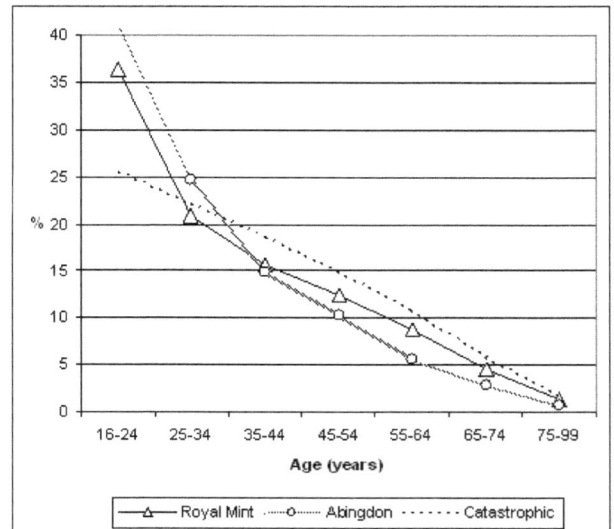

Figure 3: The sites exhibiting a catastrophic mortality distribution when age is estimated from the pubic symphyses using a catastrophic prior.

The site of Abingdon exhibits a very similar age distribution to the Royal Mint site. This was an unexpected finding, as Abingdon was not thought to be anything other than an attritional cemetery (Leeds and Harden 1936). What has led to a catastrophic age-at-death distribution amongst the adults akin to that of a plague site? The burial context does little to aid interpretation in the sense that it is not exceptional for a site of this date and location. A previous examination of the demography of the site using a different methodology did not pick up any unusual mortality profile (Gowland 2002). It is possible that this mortality pattern is the result of a particularly biased sample of pubic symphyses, however, the proportion surviving at this site is similar to that of the other cemeteries. A brief assessment of the pathological evidence by the first author provided no indication of inter-personal violence – a possible explanation for this mortality profile. A satisfactory explanation for this anomaly clearly requires further investigation into the nature of this cemetery site (Gowland in prep).

Known Age Test

One can only really provide a test of an ageing method by applying it to a skeletal series of known age individuals, distinct from the reference series on which it was based. This test has been carried out using the Brooks and Suchey (1990) reference series of 273 female individuals. Despite females being the most notoriously difficult and variable individuals to age using the pubic symphysis, Figure 4 demonstrates that the method works well. The female reference series is unlike a 'normal' attritional sample and is more akin to a catastrophic sample. This is because the Suchey-Brooks reference series was obtained from autopsy cases, many of which were homicides, suicides and accidents (Suchey et al. 1986: 40). Samples of violent adult deaths tend to generate catastrophic profiles because age-specific risks of violent death are relatively uniform.

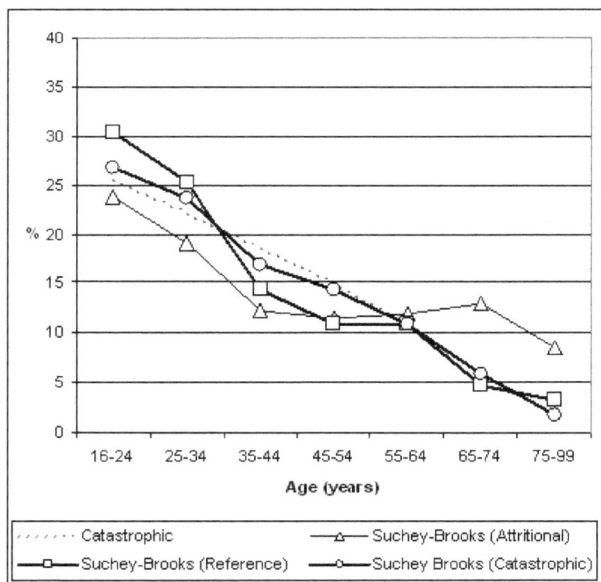

Figure 4: Test of the Bayesian pubic symphysis method on the Suchey-Brooks reference sample for females.

Figure 4 illustrates that when using either attritional or catastrophic prior probabilities the method is able to produce a good approximation of the actual mortality distribution of the reference sample. Clearly the results are improved when a catastrophic prior is used, because the catastrophic prior approximates very closely the age

structure of the Suchey-Brooks reference sample.

Conclusions

Our ability to accurately determine the mortality profiles of skeletal samples has been under serious doubt over the last two decades. As one of the primary methods of age estimation, the pubic symphysis has frequently been at the heart of attempts to produce accurate and reliable age estimation. We believe that the results discussed above, incorporating Bayesian statistics into a pubic symphyseal method, present a very encouraging indication that archaeologists can in fact produce valid approximations of the mortality distributions of past populations. When applied to the various, diverse, archaeological samples, the method produced distinctive age distributions, which (with the exception of Abingdon) accorded with the mortality distributions that one would expect given the available contextual information. The similarity between the catastrophic and attritional sites with the model age distributions is remarkable given the potential biases in skeletal preservation (e.g. Walker et al. 1988; Paine & Harpending 1998). The test of the method against an independent known age sample also indicated that the method produces reliable results. We believe that this paper has demonstrated that archaeologists can produce valid mortality distributions from cemetery populations and have confidence that the patterns that they observe are real and can be interpreted accordingly. Future production of mortality profiles, must, however, incorporate Bayesian statistics otherwise they will continue to reproduce biases in methodology.

Acknowledgements

The skeletal data were collected when Rebecca Gowland was funded by an AHRB Innovation Award (Grant number:B/IA/AN866/APN13721). Thanks are due to John Shepherd and Bill White for facilitating access to the Royal Mint skeletons and to Eugenia Cunha and Louise Humphrey for allowing us to use the Coimbra and Spitalfields known age skeletal collections.

Literature Cited

Acsádi G and Nemeskéri, J (1970) *History of Human Lifespan and Mortality*. Budapest: Akademiai Kiado.

Aykroyd RG, Lucy D, Pollard AM, and Solheim T (1997) Technical note: regression analysis in adult age estimation. *American Journal of Physical Anthropology*, 104: 259-265.

Bocquet-Appel J-P and Masset C (1982) Farewell to palaeodemography. *Journal of Human Evolution* 11: 321-333.

Bocquet-Appel J-P and Masset C (1985) Palaeodemography: resurrection or ghost? *Journal of Human Evolution* 14: 107-111.

Bocquet-Appel J-P and Masset C (1996) Paleodemography: expectancy and false hope. American *Journal of Physical Anthropology* 99: 571-583.

Boldsen, JL, Milner GR, Konigsberg LW, and Wood JW (2002) Transition analysis: a new method for estimating age from skeletons. In RD Hoppa and JW Vaupel (eds.): *Paleodemography*. Cambridge: Cambridge University Press; 73-106.

Brooks ST (1955) Skeletal age at death: the reliability of cranial and pubic age indicators. *American Journal of Physical Anthropology* 13: 567-597.

Brooks ST and Suchey JM (1990) Skeletal age determination based on the os pubis: a comparison of the Acsádi-Nemeskéri and Suchey-Brooks methods. *Human Evolution* 5: 227-238.

Chamberlain AT (2000) Problems and prospects in palaeodemography. In M Cox and S Mays (eds.): Human Osteology in Archaeology and Forensic Science. London: *Greenwich Medical Media*; 101-115.

Coale AJ and Demeny P (1983) *Regional Model Life Tables and Stable Populations* (2nd edition). Princeton: Princeton University Press.

Gelman A, Carlin JB, Stern HS, and Rubin DB (1995) *Bayesian Data Analysis*. London: Chapman and Hall.

Gilbert BM (1973) Misapplication to females of the standard for aging the male os pubis. *American Journal of Physical Anthropology* 38: 39-40.

Gilbert BM and McKern TW (1973) A method for aging the female os pubis. *American Journal of Physical Anthropology* 38: 31-38.

Gowland RL (2002) *Age as an Aspect of Social Identity in Fourth to Sixth Century AD England: The Archaeological Funerary Evidence*. Unpublished PhD, University of Durham.

Gowland RL (in preparation) *Beyond ethnicity: symbols of identity in late Roman and early Saxon Oxfordshire*.

Gowland RL and Chamberlain AT (2002) A Bayesian approach to aging perinatal skeletal material from archaeological sites: implications for the evidence for infanticide in Roman-Britain. *Journal of Archaeological Science* 29: 677-685.

Gowland RL and Chamberlain AT (in press) Detecting plague: Palaeodemographic characterisation of a catastrophic death assemblage. *Antiquity*.

Grainger I and Hawkins D (1988) Excavations at the Royal Mint site 1986-1988. *The London Archaeologist* 5: 429-436.

Hanihara K and Suzuki T (1978) Estimation of age from the pubic symphysis by means of multiple regression analysis. *American Journal of Physical Anthropology* 48: 233-240.

Hoppa RD (2000) Population variation in osteological aging criteria: an example from the pubic symphysis. *American Journal of Physical Anthropology* 111: 185-191.

Hoppa RD and Sitchon M (2003) Digital imaging of the pubic symphysis: a comparison of 2-D and 3-D approaches to assessing age-related changes. *American Journal of Physical Anthropology* 36: 117.

Hoppa RD and Vaupel JW (2002) The Rostock Manifesto for paleodemography: the way from age to stage. In RD Hoppa and JW Vaupel (eds.): *Paleodemography: Age Distributions from Skeletal Samples*. Cambridge: Cambridge University Press; 1-8.

Katz D and Suchey JM (1989) Race differences in pubic symphyseal aging patterns in the male. *American Journal of Physical Anthropology* 80: 167-172.

Keckler CNW (1997) Catastrophic mortality in simulations of forager age-at-death: where did all the humans go? In RR Paine (ed.): *Integrating Archaeological Demography: Multidisciplinary Approaches to Prehistoric Populations*. Occasional Paper No. 24. Center for Archaeological Investigations, Southern Illinois University, Carbondale; 205-228.

Klepinger LL, Katz D, Micozzi MS, and Carroll L (1992) Evaluation of cast methods for estimating age from the os pubis. *Journal of Forensic Sciences* 37: 763-770.

Konigsberg LW and Frankenberg SR (1992) Estimation of age structure in anthropological demography. *American Journal of Physical Anthropology* 89: 235-256.

Leeds ET and Harden DB (1936) *The Anglo-Saxon Cemetery at Abingdon, Berks*. Ashmolean Museum, Oxford.

Margerison BJ and Knüsel C.J (2002) Paleodemographic comparison of a catastrophic and an attritional death assemblage. *American Journal of Physical Anthropology* 119: 134-143.

Mays S (2003) Comment on 'A Bayesian approach to ageing perinatal skeletal material from archaeological sites: implications for the evidence for infanticide in Roman Britain' by R.L. Gowland and A.T. Chamberlain. *Journal of Archaeological Science* 30: 1695-1700.

McKern TW and Stewart TD (1957) *Skeletal changes in young American males.* Natick, MA: Quartermaster Research and Development Command.

Meindl RS and Lovejoy CO (1989) Age changes in the pelvis: implications for paleodemography. In MY İşcan (ed.): *Age Markers in the Human Skeleton.* Springfield: Charles C. Thomas; 137-168.

Meindl RS, Lovejoy CO, Mensforth RP, and Walker RA (1985) A revised method of age determination using the os pubis, with a review and tests of accuracy of other current methods of pubic symphysis ageing. *American Journal of Physical Anthropology* 68: 29-46.

Meindl RS and Russell KF (1998) Recent advances in method and theory in paleodemography. *Annual Review of Anthropology* 27: 375-399.

Meindl RS, Russell KF, and Lovejoy CO (1990) Reliability of age at death in the Hamann-Todd collection: validity of subselection procedures used in blind tests of the summary age technique. *American Journal of Physical Anthropology* 83: 349-357.

Molleson T and Cox M (1993) *The Spitalfields Project Volume 2. The Anthropology. The Middling Sort.* York: C.B.A. Research Report 86.

Nemeskéri J, Harsányi L, and Acsádi G (1960) Methoden zur Diagnose des Lebensalters von Skelettfunden. *Anthropologischer Anzeiger* 24: 70-95.

Paine RR (2000) If a population crashes in Prehistory, and there is no paleodemographer there to hear it, does it make a sound? *American Journal of Physical Anthropology* 112: 181-190.

Paine RR and Harpending HC (1998) Effect of sample bias on palaeodemographic fertility estimates. *American Journal of Physical Anthropology* 105: 231-240.

Pasquier E, Pernot LDM, Burdin V, Mounayer C, Le Rest C, Colin D, Mottier D, Roux C, and Baccino E (1999). Determination of age at death: assessment of an algorithm of age prediction using numerical three-dimensional CT data from pubic bones. *American Journal of Physical Anthropology* 108: 261-268.

Phillips LD (1973) *Bayesian Statistics for Social scientists.* London: Nelson.

Saunders SR, Fitzgerald C, Rogers T, Dudar JC, and McKillop H (1992) A test of several methods of skeletal age estimation using a documented archaeological sample. *Canadian Journal of Forensic Sciences* 25: 97-118.

Schmitt A (2004) Age-at-death assessment using the os pubis and the auricular surface of the ilium: a test on an identified Asian sample. *International Journal of Osteoarchaeology* 14: 1-6.

Schmitt A, Murail P, Cunha E, and Rouge D (2002) Variability of the pattern of aging on the human skeleton: evidence from bone indicators and implications on age at death estimation. *Journal of Forensic Sciences* 47: 1203-1209.

Stewart TD (1957) Distortion of the pubic symphyseal face in females and its effect on age determination. *American Journal of Physical Anthropology* 15: 9-18.

Suchey JM (1979) Problems in the ageing of females using the os pubis. *American Journal of Physical Anthropology* 51: 467-470.

Suchey JM, Wisely DV, and Katz D (1986) Evaluation of the Todd and McKern-Stewart methods for aging the male os pubis. In K Reichs (ed.): *Forensic Osteology: Advances in the Identification of Human Remains.* Springfield, Charles C. Thomas; 33-67.

Todd TW (1920) Age changes in the pubic bone: I. The Male white pubis. *American Journal of Physical Anthropology* 3: 285-334.

Todd TW (1921a) Age changes in the pubic bone: II. The pubis of the male Negro-White hybrid. *American Journal of Physical Anthropology* 4: 1-26.

Todd TW (1921b) Age changes in the pubic bone: III. The pubis of the white female. *American Journal of Physical Anthropology* 4: 26-39.

Walker PL, Johnson JR and Lambert PM (1988) Age and sex biases in the preservation of human skeletal remains. *American Journal of Physical Anthropology* 76: 183-188.

Postscript

Sonia R. Zakrzewski & Margaret Clegg

Centre for the Archaeology of Human Origins
Dept of Archaeology, University of Southampton,
Highfield, Southampton, SO17 1BF

The current volume represents the first publication of the conference proceedings of the British Association for Biological Anthropology and Osteoarchaeology and consists of a sample of the papers and posters presented at the Association's Fifth annual conference. It is hoped that this volume will therefore be the first of many. The papers presented here have demonstrated the diversity and depth of research in biological anthropology that was presented at the conference, and show the strength of the field within Archaeology and Anthropology.

We should like to thank all those who presented their research at the conference, be it in podium presentation or poster format. We would also like to thank the reviewers for their help. We also thank Carina Buckley and Sarah Clegg for their help in editing the final volume. Lastly, but by no means least, we thank all the authors for their support and understanding. We hope that this volume will be a testament to their research.

www.ingramcontent.com/pod-product-compliance
Lightning Source LLC
Chambersburg PA
CBHW061000030426
42334CB00033B/3301